CNA

FOR ALL

Arsene Junior Joseph and Rose Andree Marjorie Tocel

Table of Contents

Foreword

As we stand on the threshold of a new era in healthcare, the role of Certified Nursing Assistants (CNAs) has never been more vital. "CNA for All" represents a significant milestone in the journey of healthcare professionals, offering an invaluable resource that honors the dedication, compassion, and essential contributions of CNAs.

This book emerges at a time when the world is recognizing the significance of CNAs, the unsung heroes who work tirelessly to provide high-quality care to individuals in need. With "CNA for All," we embark on a journey through the heart and soul of healthcare, exploring the multifaceted responsibilities, challenges, and rewards that come with being a Certified Nursing Assistant.

The journey begins with an exploration of the historical evolution of the CNA role, highlighting how it has evolved into the essential position it is today. From the fundamental qualifications and certification requirements to the ethical and legal considerations that underpin CNA practice, this book provides a comprehensive foundation upon which every CNA can build their career.

Effective communication, infection control, and safe patient transfers are among the essential skills discussed, empowering CNAs to provide optimal care. Chapters on patient care, vital signs monitoring, and assisting with medication administration equip CNAs with the knowledge and tools they need to excel in their roles.

"CNA for All" does not just focus on the clinical aspects of the profession. It delves into the heart of patient care, emphasizing the importance of empathy, compassion, and emotional support. It also addresses the unique challenges of caring for special populations, such as pediatric and geriatric patients, and those with disabilities.

The book recognizes the emotional toll that the CNA role can sometimes take and offers guidance on self-care, mental health, and recognizing and addressing substance abuse and addiction issues that may arise in the healthcare setting.

As healthcare becomes increasingly diverse, "CNA for All" underscores the importance of cultural competence and respect for diversity in delivering patient-centered care. It also highlights the opportunities for professional development and career advancement available to CNAs.

Ethical dilemmas, quality improvement, and the role of CNAs in interdisciplinary collaboration are explored, offering a deeper understanding of the complex dynamics of healthcare. The book also addresses timely topics such as infection control during pandemics and the care of patients with dementia.

Through "CNA for All," CNAs will gain insights into legal and ethical considerations in end-of-life care, as well as practical guidance for assisting with activities of daily living and providing care in home and community settings.

Patient safety and error reporting are central to the CNA role, and this book empowers CNAs to champion a culture of safety and continuous improvement. Looking ahead, "CNA for All" touches on future trends that will shape the profession and offers reflections on the evolving role of CNAs in healthcare.

In closing, "CNA for All" is not just a book; it is a tribute to the dedication of CNAs and their enduring commitment to the well-being of patients. It is a guide, a mentor, and a source of inspiration for those embarking on their journey in the healthcare field.

We extend our deepest gratitude to CNAs worldwide for their unwavering dedication and resilience. We hope this book serves as a beacon, illuminating the path to excellence in CNA practice. Let it be a testament to the fact that, truly, CNAs are healthcare heroes for all.

Arsene Junior Joseph

Acknowledgments

In the journey of creating this book, I am humbled and filled with gratitude for the invaluable support and inspiration I have received from many.

First and foremost, I want to express my deepest gratitude to Jesus Christ. His boundless love, guidance, and grace have been the cornerstone of my life and the driving force behind this book. Without His presence and unwavering support, this endeavor would not have been possible.

To my beloved husband, Arsene Junior Joseph, I owe a debt of thanks that words can hardly express. Your unwavering love, constant encouragement, and profound understanding have been my greatest sources of strength throughout this endeavor. Your unwavering faith in both me and this project has served as an enduring wellspring of inspiration.

I extend my heartfelt appreciation to my dear mother, Dieula Silne Tocel, whose invaluable encouragement, and prayers have enriched the pages of this book. Your wisdom and unwavering support have been a guiding light.

I am also grateful for the technology that made this project possible, enabling me to bring my words to life.

To all those who have supported and believed in me along this journey, whether mentioned here or not, your presence and contributions have been deeply appreciated. Thank you all for being part of this remarkable journey.

For Whom Is This Book?

The book **"CNA for All"** is primarily intended for a diverse audience of individuals who are interested in or currently pursuing a career as Certified Nursing Assistants (CNAs) in the healthcare industry. This book is designed to provide comprehensive guidance, knowledge, and resources to CNAs at all stages of their careers, including:

Aspiring CNAs: Those who are considering a career as CNAs and want to learn about the profession, its responsibilities, and the requirements for certification.

Current CNAs: CNAs who are already certified and working in healthcare settings but wish to enhance their skills, knowledge, and understanding of their role to provide better patient care.

CNA Students: Individuals enrolled in CNA training programs, whether in educational institutions or online courses, looking for a supplementary resource to support their learning and prepare for certification.

Healthcare Educators: Instructors and educators who teach CNA training programs can use this book as a valuable textbook or reference material for their students.

Healthcare Managers and Employers: Administrators, nurse managers, and healthcare employers can benefit from this book to understand the essential skills, competencies, and ethical considerations required of CNAs in their organizations.

Allied Healthcare Professionals: Professionals working in allied healthcare fields, such as nurses, medical assistants, or therapists, may find this book valuable for understanding the roles and collaborations involving CNAs in healthcare teams.

Patients and Families: While not the primary audience, patients and their families can gain insights into the role of CNAs, helping them better understand the care provided by these professionals and fostering communication and collaboration in healthcare settings.

The book aims to serve as a comprehensive resource that covers various aspects of the CNA role, from fundamental skills and clinical knowledge to ethical considerations, cultural competence, and career development. It provides a foundation for CNAs to excel in their roles and contribute to the well-being of patients across diverse healthcare settings.

Introduction

In the ever-evolving landscape of healthcare, the role of Certified Nursing Assistants (CNAs) stands as an essential pillar of patient care. These dedicated professionals are the compassionate and capable hands that provide comfort, support, and vital assistance to individuals in need. As we embark on a journey through the pages of "CNA for All," we invite you to explore the multifaceted world of CNAs—a world where skill, compassion, and dedication intersect to make a profound difference in the lives of countless patients.

The heart of healthcare beats with the rhythm of countless CNAs who commit themselves daily to the well-being and comfort of those they serve. Whether in hospitals, nursing homes, assisted living facilities, or home care settings, CNAs are the unsung heroes who bridge the gap between patients and the healthcare system. This book is a tribute to their unwavering commitment.

The Role of Certified Nursing Assistants

Chapter by chapter, "CNA for All" will take you on a comprehensive journey, exploring the history, qualifications, ethical considerations, and responsibilities of CNAs. From the foundational principles of infection control to the intricacies of providing emotional support, we will delve into the skills, knowledge, and attitudes that define the CNA profession.

The scope of this book is not limited to clinical skills alone; it extends into the realm of cultural competence, diversity, and the ethical dilemmas that may arise in the course of patient care. As the healthcare landscape continues to evolve, so too does the role of CNAs. "CNA for All" offers insights into the future trends and advancements that will shape the profession, ensuring CNAs are well-prepared for the challenges and opportunities ahead.

A Source of Inspiration and Education

Whether you are an aspiring CNA, a current practitioner seeking to enhance your skills, a healthcare educator, or an allied healthcare professional, this book is tailored to provide you with the knowledge and resources needed to excel in the field of Certified Nursing Assistance.

As we explore the chapters that follow, we will uncover the complexities and rewards of CNA practice. We will emphasize the importance of not only clinical proficiency but also the qualities of empathy, compassion, and cultural sensitivity that define exceptional patient care.

A Tribute to Healthcare Heroes

Above all, "CNA for All" pays homage to the remarkable individuals who don the CNA uniform each day. It is a testament to your dedication, resilience, and unwavering commitment to the well-being of those in your care. You are the cornerstone of healthcare, and your contributions deserve the utmost recognition.

As we embark on this educational journey together, may "CNA for All" serve as a beacon, illuminating the path to excellence in CNA practice. Let it be a reminder that CNAs are indeed healthcare heroes for all.

Arsene Junior Joseph

Definition Of CNA

A Certified Nursing Assistant (CNA) is a respected and vital healthcare professional who has successfully completed a state-approved training program and passed a competency evaluation to obtain certification. The role of a CNA is of utmost importance within the healthcare industry, as these professionals provide essential direct patient care and support under the supervision of licensed nurses, such as Registered Nurses (RNs) or Licensed Practical Nurses (LPNs), and other healthcare professionals.

CNAs are often referred to as the backbone of healthcare due to their fundamental contributions to patient well-being. Their responsibilities encompass a wide range of tasks, all designed to ensure the comfort, safety, and overall care of patients in various healthcare settings. Some of their core duties include assisting patients with activities of daily living (ADLs), such as bathing, dressing, and feeding, monitoring and recording vital signs, documenting patient information, and providing emotional support to patients and their families during challenging times.

These dedicated professionals can be found working in diverse healthcare environments, including hospitals, nursing homes, long-term care facilities, rehabilitation centers, and even in home healthcare settings. In each of these settings, CNAs play an integral role in the interdisciplinary healthcare team, collaborating closely with nurses, physicians, therapists, and other healthcare providers to deliver comprehensive care.

A key aspect of the CNA's role is to ensure that patients maintain their dignity and quality of life, even in the face of illness or disability. They are often the individuals who spend the most time with patients, forming important bonds and relationships that contribute to the overall well-being of those in their care.

Furthermore, CNAs are trained to handle emergencies and provide basic first aid, making them valuable assets in situations where quick and effective response is crucial. Their ability to stay calm under pressure and their commitment to patient safety make them indispensable members of the healthcare team.

Chapter 1

The Role of Certified Nursing Assistants (CNAs)

In the vast realm of healthcare, there exists a unique and vital profession known as Certified Nursing Assistants (CNAs). These individuals form the backbone of patient care, providing essential support and compassion to those who require medical assistance. Chapter 1 of "CNA for All" delves into the multifaceted role of CNAs, highlighting their significance in the healthcare system, exploring the historical evolution of their profession, and offering real-life examples that illustrate the impact they have on patients' lives.

The Significance of CNAs in Healthcare

CNAs are healthcare professionals trained to provide direct care to patients under the supervision of registered nurses (RNs) or licensed practical nurses (LPNs). Their role is diverse and indispensable, encompassing various tasks that ensure the well-being and comfort of patients. CNAs assist with activities of daily living (ADLs), monitor vital signs, offer emotional support, and play a pivotal role in infection control.

Consider Sarah, a 78-year-old woman recovering from hip surgery at a rehabilitation center. She relies on her CNA, Mark, for assistance with bathing, dressing, and transferring from her bed to a wheelchair. Mark's gentle and attentive care not only helps Sarah regain her physical strength but also provides emotional reassurance during her challenging recovery.

The Historical Evolution of CNAs

To appreciate the significance of CNAs in contemporary healthcare, it's essential to understand their historical evolution. The roots of nursing assistance can be traced back to the early 20th century when healthcare facilities began recognizing the need for dedicated individuals to support nurses in patient care. Over time, formal training programs and certification processes emerged, shaping CNAs into the professionals they are today.

Imagine the early 1900s when healthcare institutions were predominantly staffed by nurses with limited support. Patient care was a challenging endeavor until CNAs started to bridge the gap, enabling more comprehensive care delivery. This historical perspective underscores how CNAs have grown from auxiliary roles into indispensable contributors to healthcare teams.

Examples of CNA Responsibilities

CNAs wear many hats in healthcare settings, each representing a vital aspect of patient care. Some of the core responsibilities include:

1. **Assistance with ADLs**: CNAs assist patients with activities such as bathing, dressing, toileting, and eating. They ensure that patients maintain their dignity and independence to the greatest extent possible.

For instance, John, a CNA working in a long-term care facility, helps residents like Mary with Alzheimer's disease with their daily routines. Mary may not always remember her name, but John's warm and patient assistance allows her to maintain a sense of self.

2. **Vital Signs Monitoring**: CNAs routinely measure and record vital signs like temperature, pulse, respiration rate, and blood pressure. These measurements provide crucial data for assessing patients' overall health.

Consider the case of Emily, a CNA in a busy hospital. She diligently checks and records vital signs for patients in the medical-surgical unit. Her accurate monitoring helps the medical team identify any deviations from normal ranges promptly.

3. **Emotional Support**: Beyond physical care, CNAs offer emotional support to patients who may be dealing with illness, pain, or emotional distress. They listen, provide companionship, and offer a comforting presence.

Take the example of James, a CNA in a hospice care facility. He spends time with terminally ill patients like Maria, offering a listening ear and a comforting hand. James's empathetic approach brings solace to Maria and her family during their difficult journey.

4. **Infection Control**: CNAs play a crucial role in infection control by practicing proper hand hygiene, wearing personal protective equipment (PPE), and following isolation protocols when necessary.

In a recent example during the COVID-19 pandemic, CNAs like Lisa became frontline warriors, meticulously adhering to infection control guidelines to protect vulnerable residents in long-term care facilities from the virus.

In these examples, we witness the profound impact of CNAs on patient care. They are not just healthcare providers; they are advocates for dignity, comfort, and compassion.

As we delve deeper into the chapters that follow, we will explore the educational requirements, certification processes, and ethical considerations that define the CNA profession. We will also delve into the essential communication skills that CNAs must possess to excel in their roles and ensure the best possible care for their patients.

Chapter 2

Historical Evolution of the CNA Role

The journey of Certified Nursing Assistants (CNAs) in the realm of healthcare is a compelling story of transformation and growth. Chapter 2 of "CNA for All" takes us on a historical odyssey, tracing the origins of nursing assistants, examining the development of certification programs, and shedding light on the modernization of the CNA role. Through a tapestry of historical accounts and real-world examples, we gain a deeper appreciation for how CNAs have become the essential healthcare professionals they are today.

Origins of Nursing Assistants

The roots of nursing assistance can be found in the early 20th century when the demand for dedicated individuals to support nurses in patient care began to emerge. The challenges of caring for patients in healthcare facilities became increasingly evident, leading to the recognition of the need for auxiliary personnel.

In the early days, nursing assistants were often referred to as "orderlies" or "nurse aides." These roles were predominantly filled by individuals with limited formal training but a strong commitment to patient care. They helped with basic tasks and provided crucial support to nurses.

One striking example from the early 1900s is the story of Emma, a compassionate woman who volunteered as an orderly during World War I. Emma's dedication and tireless efforts in tending to wounded soldiers showcased the potential of nursing assistants to complement the work of nurses in challenging healthcare environments.

Development of Certification Programs

As the demand for nursing assistants grew, so did the need for standardized training and certification programs. This led to the establishment of formal education and evaluation processes for aspiring CNAs. The introduction of

Certification Examinations

Upon completion of the training program, aspiring CNAs must demonstrate their competency by passing a state-approved certification examination. These exams typically consist of two parts: a written or computer-based knowledge test and a skills evaluation performed in a clinical setting.

Consider the experience of Alex, who diligently studied the material covered in his training program and practiced the necessary skills under the guidance of experienced instructors. When the day of the certification exam arrived, Alex approached it with confidence. He completed the written portion successfully, showcasing his understanding of theoretical concepts. In the skills evaluation, he demonstrated his ability to perform tasks such as assisting with bathing, taking vital signs, and providing emotional support to a simulated patient.

Alex's journey underscores the significance of certification examinations in assessing the competence of CNAs. These exams serve as a standardized measure of a CNA's knowledge and ability to provide safe and effective patient care.

Continuing Education for CNAs

Certification is not the end of a CNA's educational journey; it is the beginning of a commitment to lifelong learning and professional development. Continuing education is essential for CNAs to stay current with advances in healthcare, refresh their skills, and expand their knowledge.

Consider the example of Sarah, a seasoned CNA with years of experience in a long-term care facility. Sarah recognizes the importance of staying up-to-date with the latest techniques and best practices in patient care. She regularly attends workshops and seminars on topics such as dementia care, pain management, and cultural competence. Sarah's dedication to continuing education not only benefits her professional growth but also enhances the quality of care she provides to her residents.

Chapter 4

Ethical and Legal Considerations

The role of a Certified Nursing Assistant (CNA) in healthcare is not only defined by clinical skills but also by a profound commitment to ethical and legal principles. Chapter 4 of "CNA for All" explores the ethical code that guides CNAs, delves into their legal responsibilities and boundaries, and emphasizes the critical importance of reporting and documentation. Real-life examples and scenarios illustrate how CNAs navigate complex ethical and legal dilemmas in their daily practice.

Code of Ethics for CNAs

Ethical principles form the moral compass that guides CNAs in providing patient-centered care. A fundamental aspect of their role is adhering to a code of ethics that outlines their responsibilities and expectations. The principles of beneficence (doing good), non-maleficence (avoiding harm), autonomy (respecting patient choices), and justice (fairness) serve as the foundation for ethical practice.

Imagine Sarah, a CNA working in a hospice care facility. She cares for a terminally ill patient named Mr. Johnson, who expresses his desire to spend his final moments at home. Sarah, guided by the principles of autonomy and beneficence, advocates for Mr. Johnson's wish and collaborates with the healthcare team to arrange for his transfer home. Her commitment to honoring patient preferences reflects the ethical underpinning of CNA practice.

Legal Responsibilities and Boundaries

While ethical principles guide CNAs' moral decisions, the legal framework establishes the boundaries within which they must operate. CNAs are responsible for understanding the laws and regulations that govern their practice, ensuring that they provide care within the limits of their scope of practice.

Consider the case of David, a CNA providing care to a patient with a complex medical condition. While David is skilled in assisting with activities of daily living and monitoring vital signs, he recognizes that administering medications is beyond his scope of practice. Instead of attempting to do so, he promptly informs the nurse in charge, ensuring that the patient receives the appropriate medication from a licensed professional. This exemplifies how CNAs maintain their legal boundaries while prioritizing patient safety.

Reporting and Documentation

Accurate and timely reporting and documentation are crucial aspects of CNA practice. CNAs are often the eyes and ears of the healthcare team, observing and recording vital information about patients' conditions. Clear and thorough documentation helps in maintaining continuity of care, monitoring changes in patient status, and ensuring accountability.

Imagine Emily, a CNA working in a busy hospital ward. She notices that one of her patients, Mrs. Anderson, is experiencing increased pain and discomfort. Emily immediately notifies the nurse and documents the specifics of Mrs. Anderson's condition, including the time of the report. This documentation serves as a crucial record of the patient's needs and the actions taken by the healthcare team.

Complex Ethical Dilemmas

In the course of their practice, CNAs may encounter complex ethical dilemmas that require careful consideration and decision-making. These dilemmas can involve issues such as end-of-life care, informed consent, and conflicts between a patient's wishes and medical recommendations.

Consider the scenario of Mark, a CNA caring for a patient with a life-limiting illness who has expressed a desire to discontinue life-sustaining treatments. Mark faces the ethical dilemma of respecting the patient's autonomy while also considering the potential impact on the patient's family.

Chapter 5

Communication Skills for CNAs

Effective communication lies at the heart of quality patient care. Chapter 5 of "CNA for All" explores the essential role of communication skills in the practice of Certified Nursing Assistants (CNAs). Through real-life examples, practical insights, and in-depth discussions, we delve into the nuances of effective verbal and non-verbal communication, emphasizing the importance of interacting with patients and healthcare teams with empathy and professionalism.

Effective Verbal Communication

Verbal communication is a cornerstone of CNA practice, as it enables CNAs to convey information, provide reassurance, and establish rapport with patients. Clear and respectful communication is essential for ensuring patient understanding and comfort.

Consider the case of John, a CNA caring for a post-operative patient named Susan. Susan is anxious about her upcoming surgery, and John recognizes the importance of addressing her concerns. He sits down with Susan, maintains eye contact, and uses simple, non-medical language to explain the procedure and answer her questions. John's effective verbal communication not only alleviates Susan's anxiety but also empowers her to actively participate in her care decisions.

Non-Verbal Communication

Non-verbal communication encompasses body language, facial expressions, gestures, and tone of voice. CNAs must be attuned to these cues, as they can convey emotions, comfort, and empathy to patients. Conversely, misinterpreted non-verbal signals can lead to misunderstandings or anxiety.

Imagine Emily, a CNA attending to an elderly resident named Mr. Rodriguez. While Mr. Rodriguez has difficulty communicating verbally due to a recent stroke, Emily understands the importance of non-verbal cues. She maintains a warm smile, maintains eye contact, and uses gentle touch to convey her empathy and support. Through these non-verbal signals, Emily establishes a strong connection with Mr. Rodriguez, enhancing his sense of security and well-being.

Interacting with Patients and Healthcare Teams

CNAs serve as a bridge between patients and the broader healthcare team, making effective communication with both groups crucial. CNAs must listen attentively to patients, report changes in their condition accurately, and collaborate seamlessly with nurses, physicians, and other healthcare professionals.

Consider the scenario of Sarah, a CNA working in a long-term care facility. She observes that one of her residents, Mr. Thompson, is displaying signs of discomfort. Sarah promptly reports her observations to the nurse in charge and provides detailed information about Mr. Thompson's condition. Her clear and concise communication ensures that Mr. Thompson receives the necessary attention from the healthcare team, facilitating timely intervention and improving his comfort.

In healthcare settings, teamwork is paramount, and CNAs play a pivotal role in interdisciplinary collaboration. Effective communication with nurses and other team members fosters a collaborative environment where patient care is optimized. CNAs like Mark, who engage in open and respectful dialogue with their colleagues, contribute to the seamless coordination of care and better patient outcomes.

Challenges in Communication

While effective communication is a cornerstone of CNA practice, it can present challenges. CNAs may encounter patients with communication barriers due to language differences, hearing impairment, or cognitive deficits.

Chapter 6

Assisting with Activities of Daily Living (ADLs)

One of the primary responsibilities of Certified Nursing Assistants (CNAs) is to assist patients with activities of daily living (ADLs). These fundamental tasks are essential for maintaining the comfort, dignity, and overall well-being of patients. Chapter 6 of "CNA for All" delves into the intricacies of assisting with ADLs, offering real-life examples and detailed insights into how CNAs provide support in tasks ranging from bathing and dressing to toileting and feeding.

Bathing and Personal Hygiene

Bathing is a fundamental ADL that not only promotes cleanliness but also contributes to a patient's physical and emotional well-being. CNAs often assist patients with bathing, and this process requires sensitivity, respect for privacy, and attention to the patient's comfort.

Consider the experience of John, a CNA working in a rehabilitation center. He assists a patient, Mr. Williams, with a bath after a strenuous physical therapy session. John ensures the water temperature is suitable, maintains Mr. Williams' dignity by using towels to cover unexposed areas, and engages in friendly conversation to ease any discomfort. Through his thoughtful approach, John not only completes the task but also enhances Mr. Williams' sense of care and well-being.

Dressing and Grooming

Assisting patients with dressing and grooming involves more than just helping them put on clothes or comb their hair. It requires CNAs to consider the patient's preferences, limitations, and comfort. CNAs often provide valuable emotional support during this ADL, as patients may feel vulnerable during these activities.

Imagine Emily, a CNA working in a long-term care facility, assisting Mrs. Davis, a resident with limited mobility, with dressing in the morning. Emily recognizes the importance of involving Mrs. Davis in choosing her outfit and accessories, even though it may take a bit longer. This collaborative approach not only empowers Mrs. Davis but also preserves her sense of self and independence.

Toileting and Incontinence Care

Maintaining a patient's dignity and privacy while assisting with toileting and incontinence care is of utmost importance. CNAs are trained to provide respectful and sensitive assistance in this area, whether it involves helping patients use the toilet, change adult briefs, or maintain personal hygiene.

Consider the scenario of Sarah, a CNA in a nursing home, assisting Mr. Johnson, a resident with limited mobility, with toileting. Sarah ensures that Mr. Johnson's privacy is maintained, communicates clearly and respectfully, and provides emotional support throughout the process. By approaching this sensitive ADL with compassion and professionalism, Sarah helps Mr. Johnson maintain his dignity.

Feeding and Nutrition

Proper nutrition is a key element of patient care, and CNAs often play a crucial role in assisting patients with feeding. This ADL goes beyond simply serving meals; it involves ensuring that patients receive the nutrition they need while considering their dietary restrictions and preferences.

In a hospital setting, Mark, a CNA, assists Mrs. Miller, a post-surgery patient, with her meals. Mark takes the time to review Mrs. Miller's dietary restrictions and preferences, ensures the food is at an appropriate temperature, and assists her with feeding at a pace that is comfortable for her. His attention to detail and empathy enhance Mrs. Miller's overall experience and contribute to her recovery.

Chapter 7

Vital Signs Monitoring and Documentation

The ability to monitor vital signs is a core skill that sets Certified Nursing Assistants (CNAs) apart as crucial members of the healthcare team. In Chapter 7 of "CNA for All," we delve into the significance of vital signs monitoring, explore the various vital signs measured, and discuss the importance of accurate documentation. Real-life examples and practical insights illuminate how CNAs play a vital role in assessing patients' well-being through regular monitoring.

The Importance of Vital Signs

Vital signs are essential indicators of a patient's overall health and well-being. They provide critical information about the functioning of vital organs and help healthcare professionals identify deviations from normal ranges that may indicate underlying health issues.

Consider the role of Emily, a CNA in a busy hospital. She understands that regularly monitoring vital signs, such as temperature, pulse, respiration rate, and blood pressure, is a fundamental aspect of patient care. These measurements serve as valuable data points that guide clinical decisions and interventions. For example, if Emily observes a sudden increase in a patient's heart rate, she promptly reports it to the nurse, potentially leading to timely interventions and improved patient outcomes.

Temperature Monitoring

Temperature monitoring is a key vital sign that can provide valuable insights into a patient's health. CNAs often assist in measuring and recording temperatures, which can help detect fever or hypothermia.

Imagine Sarah, a CNA working in a long-term care facility. She is responsible for regularly checking the temperatures of residents. If she notices that a resident, Mr. Anderson, has an elevated temperature, she promptly reports it to the nurse. This early detection of fever allows for timely intervention and the initiation of appropriate treatment.

Pulse Assessment

Pulse assessment involves measuring the heart rate, which is a critical vital sign. CNAs are trained to locate a patient's pulse, count the beats per minute, and assess the pulse's quality and regularity.

In a skilled nursing facility, Mark, a CNA, is responsible for assessing the pulses of residents like Mrs. Johnson. He not only counts her pulse but also notes its strength and rhythm. If he detects any irregularities or significant changes, he communicates this information to the nursing team, enabling prompt evaluation and necessary interventions.

Respiration Rate Observation

Respiration rate, or the number of breaths per minute, is another vital sign closely monitored by CNAs. Changes in respiration rate can be indicative of respiratory distress or other health issues.

Consider John, a CNA in a rehabilitation center. He keeps a vigilant eye on patients' respiration rates, especially those recovering from surgery or respiratory conditions. If he observes rapid or shallow breathing in a patient, he promptly notifies the nurse. This timely communication can lead to interventions that alleviate respiratory distress.

Blood Pressure Measurement

Blood pressure is a vital sign that reflects the force of blood against the walls of the arteries. CNAs are trained to use blood pressure cuffs and stethoscopes to measure and record blood pressure accurately.

In a home care setting, Jessica, a CNA, assists a patient with hypertension in monitoring their blood pressure regularly. She ensures that the measurement is taken correctly, using appropriate techniques, and documents the readings accurately. Her diligence helps the patient and their healthcare provider manage their condition effectively.

Accurate Documentation

Accurate documentation of vital signs is essential in healthcare. CNAs play a critical role in maintaining detailed and precise records of vital sign measurements. Accurate documentation ensures that healthcare providers have access to up-to-date information that guides diagnosis and treatment.

Chapter 7 underscores that CNAs are not mere recorders of vital signs but crucial contributors to patient assessment and care planning. By mastering the art of vital signs monitoring, CNAs enhance patient safety, facilitate early detection of health issues, and contribute to improved patient outcomes.

Chapter 8

Safety Measures in Patient Care

Safety is paramount in healthcare, and Certified Nursing Assistants (CNAs) are instrumental in ensuring the well-being of patients. In Chapter 8 of "CNA for All," we explore the multifaceted role of CNAs in maintaining a safe environment for patients. Through real-life examples, detailed insights, and practical advice, we delve into infection control, fall prevention, and emergency preparedness to highlight how CNAs contribute to patient safety.

Infection Control

Infection control is a cornerstone of patient safety, and CNAs play a pivotal role in preventing the spread of infections in healthcare settings. They are trained in standard precautions, which include hand hygiene, the use of personal protective equipment (PPE), and proper disposal of contaminated materials.

Imagine Emily, a CNA in a long-term care facility, assisting a resident with dressing changes for a wound infection. She diligently follows infection control protocols, including thorough handwashing before and after the procedure, wearing gloves, and disposing of used materials in biohazard containers. Emily's commitment to infection control safeguards not only the resident's health but also the well-being of others in the facility.

Fall Prevention

Preventing falls is a crucial aspect of patient safety, particularly among elderly or mobility-impaired patients. CNAs are often at the forefront of fall prevention efforts, ensuring that patients have a safe and secure environment.

Consider Sarah, a CNA in a hospital, caring for an elderly patient, Mr. Peterson, who has a history of falls. She assesses his room for potential hazards, ensures that the call bell is within his reach, and assists him with mobility, using proper transfer techniques. Sarah's vigilance and proactive measures significantly reduce the risk of falls, enhancing Mr. Peterson's safety during his hospital stay.

Emergency Preparedness

Being prepared for emergencies is essential in healthcare, and CNAs must be well-versed in emergency response protocols. They are trained to respond quickly and effectively to various emergency situations, including fires, cardiac arrests, and medical crises.

In a skilled nursing facility, Mark, a CNA, is part of the facility's emergency response team. He knows the location of emergency equipment, such as fire extinguishers and automated external defibrillators (AEDs), and is trained to initiate cardiopulmonary resuscitation (CPR) if needed. Mark's preparedness and swift response can make a critical difference in emergency situations, potentially saving lives.

Patient Advocacy

Patient safety also involves advocacy, where CNAs act as the voice of the patient. They advocate for the rights and well-being of patients, ensuring that their concerns and preferences are heard and respected by the healthcare team.

Consider John, a CNA caring for a patient, Mrs. Davis, who is experiencing pain and discomfort. John communicates Mrs. Davis's pain to the nurse, advocating for her need for pain relief. He ensures that Mrs. Davis's pain is adequately assessed and addressed, thereby promoting her comfort and well-being.

Promoting a Culture of Safety

CNAs also contribute to promoting a culture of safety within healthcare facilities. They report safety concerns, participate in safety committees, and collaborate with colleagues to identify and address potential hazards.

Chapter 9

Dementia Care and Specialized Patient Needs

Providing care for patients with dementia and addressing specialized patient needs requires a unique set of skills and approaches. Chapter 9 of "CNA for All" explores the challenges and rewards of caring for patients with dementia and individuals with specific healthcare requirements. Real-life examples and detailed insights illustrate how CNAs play a crucial role in ensuring the comfort, dignity, and quality of life of these special patient populations.

Caring for Patients with Dementia

Patients with dementia, such as Alzheimer's disease, present distinctive challenges in healthcare. CNAs often provide care to individuals with cognitive impairments, and their approach must be tailored to meet the unique needs of these patients.

Imagine Sarah, a CNA in a memory care unit, providing care to residents with varying stages of dementia. She employs strategies like maintaining a consistent routine, using clear and simple language, and engaging residents in activities that stimulate cognitive function. Through her specialized approach, Sarah creates a supportive and comforting environment that enhances the well-being of residents.

Emotional Support for Patients with Dementia

Emotional support is a vital aspect of caring for patients with dementia. CNAs must possess empathy, patience, and effective communication skills to connect with these individuals and address their emotional needs.

In a long-term care facility, Mark, a CNA, cares for Mr. Johnson, a resident with advanced dementia who often experiences confusion and anxiety. Mark uses a calm and reassuring tone when interacting with Mr. Johnson, offering a comforting presence and validation of his feelings. By providing emotional support, Mark helps ease Mr. Johnson's distress and improve his overall quality of life.

Specialized Patient Needs

Patients with specific healthcare requirements, such as those with disabilities, chronic conditions, or unique cultural backgrounds, may necessitate specialized care. CNAs are trained to adapt their approach to meet these diverse needs.

Consider Emily, a CNA providing care for a patient with a physical disability. She collaborates with the patient to create a care plan that ensures their comfort and independence. Emily's willingness to accommodate the patient's specific needs, such as using assistive devices or adjusting the environment, promotes the patient's overall well-being and quality of life.

Palliative and End-of-Life Care

CNAs are also instrumental in providing palliative and end-of-life care, which requires a compassionate and empathetic approach. They support patients with life-limiting illnesses and their families, focusing on pain management, comfort, and emotional well-being.

In a hospice care facility, John, a CNA, cares for terminally ill patients like Maria. He provides emotional support to Maria and her family, ensuring that her final moments are filled with dignity and comfort. John's compassionate care and presence help ease the burden of a difficult journey for the patient and her loved ones.

Chapter 9 emphasizes that CNAs are versatile healthcare professionals capable of adapting to the unique needs of patients with dementia and those with specialized healthcare requirements. By providing specialized care, emotional support, and dignity to these individuals, CNAs play a pivotal role in enhancing their quality of life and ensuring that their specific needs are met with compassion and professionalism.

Chapter 10

Assisting with Mobility and Rehabilitation

Assisting patients with mobility and participating in their rehabilitation processes are integral aspects of the Certified Nursing Assistant (CNA) role. In Chapter 10 of "CNA for All," we explore the importance of maintaining and promoting patients' physical well-being through activities such as transferring, ambulation, and rehabilitation exercises. Real-life examples and detailed insights illustrate how CNAs contribute to enhancing patients' mobility and overall recovery.

Transferring Patients Safely

Transferring patients safely from one surface to another, such as from a bed to a chair, is a fundamental skill for CNAs. The goal is to prevent injuries to both the patient and the caregiver while maintaining the patient's comfort and dignity.

Imagine Emily, a CNA working in a rehabilitation center, assisting Mr. Johnson, a post-surgery patient, with transferring from his bed to a wheelchair. Emily follows proper body mechanics, ensuring that her movements are smooth and controlled. She communicates clearly with Mr. Johnson throughout the process, and together, they accomplish the transfer safely and comfortably. Emily's skillful transfer techniques minimize the risk of injury and contribute to Mr. Johnson's recovery.

Ambulation and Walking Assistance

Assisting patients with ambulation, or walking, is another crucial aspect of CNA practice. Patients may require support due to mobility limitations, post-surgical conditions, or rehabilitation goals.

In a long-term care facility, Mark, a CNA, helps Mrs. Davis, a resident recovering from a hip fracture, regain her walking ability. Mark provides physical support while ensuring Mrs. Davis maintains her balance and stability.

He encourages her with positive reinforcement and celebrates her progress during each walking session. Mark's dedication to Mrs. Davis's mobility contributes to her regaining her independence and quality of life.

Participating in Rehabilitation

CNAs play a vital role in patients' rehabilitation processes, collaborating with physical therapists and occupational therapists to implement rehabilitation plans. Rehabilitation may involve exercises, range-of-motion activities, and functional tasks that aim to improve a patient's physical abilities.

Consider John, a CNA working in a hospital's rehabilitation unit, assisting patients like Sarah, who is recovering from a stroke. John facilitates Sarah's therapy sessions by setting up equipment, providing assistance during exercises, and tracking her progress. His active involvement in Sarah's rehabilitation plan helps her regain strength and regain functional independence.

Promoting Independence and Confidence

One of the overarching goals of assisting with mobility and rehabilitation is to promote patients' independence and confidence in their abilities. CNAs empower patients to regain control over their physical well-being, which can have a profound impact on their overall quality of life.

In a home care setting, Jessica, a CNA, assists Mr. Anderson, a patient with limited mobility, with exercises prescribed by his physical therapist. Jessica not only helps Mr. Anderson perform the exercises but also educates him on their purpose and benefits. Through her encouragement and guidance, Jessica empowers Mr. Anderson to actively participate in his recovery, fostering a sense of accomplishment and self-assurance.

Chapter 11

Understanding Cognitive Impairments and Mental Health

Cognitive impairments and mental health issues are prevalent conditions that impact many patients in healthcare settings. In Chapter 11 of "CNA for All," we explore the importance of understanding and addressing cognitive impairments, such as Alzheimer's disease and dementia, as well as mental health challenges faced by patients. Real-life examples and detailed insights illustrate how CNAs play a significant role in providing compassionate care and support to individuals with these conditions.

Understanding Cognitive Impairments

Cognitive impairments, such as Alzheimer's disease and dementia, can profoundly affect a person's memory, thinking, and behavior. CNAs often care for patients with cognitive impairments and must approach their care with patience, empathy, and specialized strategies.

Consider Sarah, a CNA in a memory care unit, providing care to residents with varying degrees of dementia. She understands the importance of creating a calming and structured environment. Sarah engages residents in activities that stimulate cognitive function, using techniques like reminiscence therapy to help residents recall pleasant memories. Through her approach, Sarah contributes to enhancing the quality of life for residents with cognitive impairments.

Supporting Patients with Mental Health Challenges

Mental health challenges, such as anxiety, depression, and bipolar disorder, are common among patients in healthcare settings. CNAs play a critical role in providing emotional support and recognizing signs of mental distress.

In a hospital ward, Mark, a CNA, cares for a patient, Emily, who is experiencing symptoms of anxiety. Mark employs active listening and empathy to help Emily express her feelings and concerns. He communicates her needs to the nursing team, ensuring that she receives appropriate mental health support. Mark's compassionate care alleviates Emily's distress and contributes to her overall well-being.

Behavioral Interventions

Caring for individuals with cognitive impairments and mental health challenges often requires employing behavioral interventions. CNAs are trained to use techniques that promote positive behaviors and manage challenging behaviors effectively.

Imagine John, a CNA in a long-term care facility, caring for Mr. Johnson, a resident with Alzheimer's disease who occasionally exhibits agitated behavior. John utilizes redirection techniques, diversional activities, and a calm demeanor to manage Mr. Johnson's challenging behaviors. Through his skillful interventions, John creates a more peaceful and comfortable environment for Mr. Johnson and the other residents.

Emotional Support and Communication

Providing emotional support and effective communication are pivotal when caring for individuals with cognitive impairments and mental health conditions. CNAs must be attuned to non-verbal cues and adapt their communication style to the patient's needs.

In a psychiatric unit, Jessica, a CNA, cares for a patient, David, who has schizophrenia. Jessica uses active listening and a non-judgmental approach when communicating with David. She acknowledges his feelings and provides reassurance. Through her empathetic and supportive communication, Jessica helps David feel more understood and valued, fostering a therapeutic relationship.

Chapter 12

End-of-Life Care and Compassion

End-of-life care is a profoundly sensitive and essential aspect of healthcare, and Certified Nursing Assistants (CNAs) play a pivotal role in providing compassionate support to patients and their families during this challenging time. In Chapter 12 of "CNA for All," we delve into the significance of end-of-life care, the principles of hospice care, and the emotional and practical aspects of accompanying patients on their final journey. Real-life examples and detailed insights illustrate how CNAs offer comfort, dignity, and support to individuals at the end of life.

Understanding End-of-Life Care

End-of-life care encompasses a range of services and interventions that aim to ensure the comfort and dignity of individuals who are facing a terminal illness or are in the final stages of their life. CNAs are an integral part of the interdisciplinary healthcare team that provides end-of-life care.

Consider Sarah, a CNA in a hospice care facility, caring for a patient named Mrs. Johnson, who has a life-limiting illness. Sarah understands the importance of addressing not only Mrs. Johnson's physical needs but also her emotional and spiritual well-being during this crucial time. Sarah's empathetic presence and attentive care provide solace to Mrs. Johnson and her family.

Principles of Hospice Care

Hospice care is a specialized approach to end-of-life care that prioritizes comfort, pain management, and quality of life for patients with terminal conditions. CNAs working in hospice settings follow the principles of hospice care, which include pain and symptom management, emotional and psychological support, and respectful end-of-life planning.

In a hospice home, Mark, a CNA, provides care to Mr. Anderson, a patient in the final stages of cancer. Mark ensures that Mr. Anderson is kept comfortable

33

through diligent pain management and symptom relief. He also engages in active listening and emotional support, allowing Mr. Anderson to express his fears and wishes. Mark's commitment to hospice principles fosters a peaceful and dignified transition for Mr. Anderson and his family.

Emotional Support for Patients and Families

End-of-life care involves not only providing physical comfort but also offering emotional support to patients and their families. CNAs often play a crucial role in being a source of comfort, a listening ear, and a compassionate presence.

Imagine John, a CNA working in a hospital's palliative care unit, caring for Maria, a patient with a life-limiting illness. John not only tends to Maria's physical needs but also engages in heartfelt conversations, allowing Maria to share her life stories and concerns. He provides comfort not only to Maria but also to her family members, who are deeply appreciative of his empathetic care.

Ensuring Dignity and Respect

Preserving the dignity and respect of patients at the end of life is paramount. CNAs are trained to provide care that upholds the patient's autonomy and choices while ensuring comfort and compassion.

In a nursing home, Jessica, a CNA, cares for Mr. Thompson, a resident in the final stages of a terminal illness. Jessica respects Mr. Thompson's choices regarding his care and engages in discussions about his preferences for pain management and end-of-life decisions. Her approach ensures that Mr. Thompson's wishes are honored, and he experiences a dignified and peaceful transition.

Chapter 13

Ethical and Cultural Competence in CNA Practice

Certified Nursing Assistants (CNAs) must navigate diverse ethical and cultural landscapes in their daily practice. Chapter 13 of "CNA for All" explores the importance of ethical decision-making and cultural competence in providing patient-centered care. Real-life examples and detailed insights illustrate how CNAs uphold ethical principles and provide culturally sensitive care to diverse patient populations.

Ethical Decision-Making

Ethical decision-making is a cornerstone of CNA practice, ensuring that patients receive care that respects their values, preferences, and rights. CNAs must be equipped to navigate complex ethical dilemmas and make decisions that prioritize patient well-being.

Consider Sarah, a CNA in a long-term care facility, who is faced with an ethical dilemma. One of her residents, Mr. Johnson, has expressed a strong desire to have his daughter, who lives out of state, visit him. However, the facility has strict visitation policies due to the ongoing pandemic. Sarah engages in open communication with the facility's administration, advocating for Mr. Johnson's emotional well-being and the importance of family connection. Her ethical decision to prioritize Mr. Johnson's emotional needs ultimately leads to a compassionate resolution that allows for safe visitation.

Respecting Patient Autonomy

Respecting patient autonomy is a fundamental ethical principle that CNAs must uphold. This principle emphasizes the importance of involving patients in decision-making about their care and respecting their right to make choices.

In a home care setting, Mark, a CNA, provides care to a patient named Mrs. Davis, who has specific dietary preferences due to cultural and religious beliefs. Mark ensures that Mrs. Davis's dietary choices are honored, and he collaborates with her to create meals that align with her cultural and dietary requirements. Mark's respect for Mrs. Davis's autonomy and cultural preferences enhances her sense of control and well-being.

Cultural Competence

Cultural competence is the ability to understand, respect, and provide care that is sensitive to the cultural backgrounds and beliefs of patients. CNAs must be culturally competent to provide care that is inclusive and respectful of diversity.

Imagine Emily, a CNA working in a multicultural long-term care facility. She cares for residents from various cultural backgrounds, including a Korean resident, Mr. Kim. Emily takes the time to learn about Mr. Kim's cultural traditions and preferences, such as his dietary choices and communication styles. By incorporating cultural competence into her care, Emily ensures that Mr. Kim feels valued and respected.

Ethical Challenges in Cultural Contexts

Ethical challenges can become more complex when they intersect with cultural beliefs and practices. CNAs must be prepared to address ethical dilemmas that arise in culturally diverse healthcare settings.

In a hospice care facility, Jessica, a CNA, cares for a terminally ill patient, Maria, from a culture that places a strong emphasis on family decision-making. Jessica faces an ethical challenge when Maria's family members have differing opinions about her end-of-life care. Jessica collaborates with the healthcare team and engages in culturally sensitive communication to navigate this complex situation. Her ability to respect cultural values while upholding ethical principles leads to a resolution that aligns with Maria's best interests.

Chapter 14

Infection Control in Healthcare

Infection control is a fundamental aspect of healthcare that directly impacts patient safety and well-being. Chapter 14 of "CNA for All" explores the critical role of Certified Nursing Assistants (CNAs) in infection control and the prevention of healthcare-associated infections (HAIs). Real-life examples and detailed insights illustrate how CNAs uphold stringent infection control practices to protect patients, themselves, and their colleagues.

Understanding Healthcare-Associated Infections (HAIs)

Healthcare-associated infections (HAIs) are infections that patients acquire while receiving medical treatment in healthcare facilities. CNAs are instrumental in preventing HAIs by adhering to strict infection control protocols.

Consider Sarah, a CNA working in a hospital's surgical ward. She understands that post-surgical patients are at risk of surgical site infections. To prevent HAIs, Sarah follows meticulous hand hygiene practices, ensures aseptic techniques during wound care, and educates patients on the importance of keeping incisions clean and dry. Her diligence in infection control reduces the risk of HAIs and contributes to positive patient outcomes.

Hand Hygiene and PPE

Hand hygiene is one of the most effective measures in preventing the spread of infections. CNAs must practice proper hand hygiene before and after every patient interaction. Additionally, the correct use of personal protective equipment (PPE), such as gloves and gowns, is crucial to protect both patients and healthcare workers.

In a long-term care facility, Mark, a CNA, provides care to residents with various healthcare needs. He demonstrates consistent hand hygiene practices, including thorough handwashing and the use of hand sanitizer. Mark also utilizes PPE when necessary, such as when assisting residents with isolation precautions. His commitment to hand hygiene and PPE use helps maintain a safe and infection-free environment.

Environmental Cleaning and Disinfection

Maintaining a clean and disinfected environment is essential to prevent the transmission of infections. CNAs must be diligent in cleaning and disinfecting frequently-touched surfaces and equipment in patient care areas.

Imagine Emily, a CNA in a rehabilitation center, where multiple patients share exercise equipment. Emily follows a rigorous cleaning and disinfection schedule, ensuring that all equipment is thoroughly cleaned after each use. Her dedication to environmental cleaning reduces the risk of cross-contamination and keeps patients safe from HAIs.

Respiratory Hygiene and Safe Practices

Respiratory hygiene is crucial in preventing the spread of respiratory infections, including influenza and respiratory viruses. CNAs must educate patients and adhere to safe practices when dealing with respiratory illnesses.

In a nursing home, Jessica, a CNA, cares for residents during flu season. She provides residents with information about respiratory hygiene, including proper cough etiquette and the importance of wearing masks when appropriate. Jessica also practices these measures herself, setting an example for both residents and staff members. Her proactive approach helps prevent the spread of respiratory infections within the facility.

Reporting and Surveillance

CNAs are often the first to observe changes in a patient's condition that may indicate an infection. Timely reporting of such changes is essential for prompt intervention and containment of potential outbreaks.

Chapter 15

Understanding CNA Field Pathologies

Certified Nursing Assistants (CNAs) are essential pillars in the realm of patient care, and their proficiency in understanding a wide array of medical conditions and pathologies is pivotal for delivering effective and compassionate care. This chapter takes an in-depth dive into the indispensable knowledge that CNAs must acquire to navigate the complexities of pathologies they may encounter throughout their healthcare careers. Through real-life scenarios and detailed insights, we will illuminate how CNAs can best comprehend, address, and provide exceptional care to patients grappling with a spectrum of medical conditions, all while upholding the highest standards of healthcare professionalism.

Building a Solid Foundation of Pathology Knowledge for CNAs

To provide exceptional care, CNAs must establish a strong foundational understanding of a multitude of medical conditions and pathologies. This knowledge empowers them to recognize symptoms, comprehend treatment plans, and offer unwavering support to patients dealing with these health challenges.

Consider Mary, an exemplary CNA working diligently in a long-term care facility. Her responsibilities encompass the care of residents with diverse medical conditions, including diabetes. Mary's profound knowledge of diabetes equips her with the ability to assist residents in monitoring their blood glucose levels, administering insulin when necessary, and promptly identifying signs of hypo- or hyperglycemia. Her expertise ensures that residents receive not just care but comprehensive, condition-specific care.

Exploring the Spectrum of Common Pathologies in CNA Practice

The path of a CNA is paved with encounters involving a wide spectrum of pathologies, from chronic conditions such as diabetes and hypertension to acute ailments like infections and injuries. An in-depth understanding of these conditions is indispensable for providing precise care and empathetic support.

In a bustling hospital setting, we meet John, a dedicated CNA who frequently tends to patients grappling with respiratory conditions like chronic obstructive pulmonary disease (COPD). John's expertise in COPD allows him to swiftly identify signs of respiratory distress, competently assist with oxygen therapy, and ensure that patients adhere rigorously to their prescribed treatment regimens. His knowledge becomes a vital link in the chain of patient care, contributing to better outcomes.

The Art of Recognizing and Responding to Symptoms

The ability to recognize and respond to symptoms is a hallmark skill for CNAs. Early detection and prompt intervention often prove to be the linchpin of positive patient outcomes.

Picture Sarah, a compassionate CNA in a rehabilitation center, providing care for a patient who recently endured a stroke. Sarah's comprehensive understanding of stroke symptoms enables her to discern potential complications, such as difficulty swallowing or muscle weakness. Her vigilant observation and quick action mean that she can promptly notify the nursing team, ensuring that the patient receives the precise care and attention needed for a smoother recovery.

Collaboration and Communication: The Cornerstone of Managing Pathologies

CNAs are integral members of the healthcare team, and effective communication and collaboration stand as non-negotiables when it comes to managing patients afflicted by complex medical conditions. CNAs must collaborate closely with nurses, physicians, and other healthcare professionals to guarantee that patients receive holistic and tailored care.

In a nurturing nursing home environment, we encounter David, a dedicated CNA who seamlessly collaborates with the nursing staff to care for residents diagnosed with Alzheimer's disease. He serves as a vital conduit of information, communicating any changes in residents' behavior or cognitive function to the healthcare team. His effective communication fosters timely adjustments to residents' care plans, ensuring their safety, well-being, and quality of life.

The Commitment to Continuous Learning and Adaptation

Pathologies and medical knowledge are dynamic, continually evolving with time. As a result, CNAs must engage in ongoing learning and adaptation to remain current with the latest developments in healthcare. This unwavering commitment to lifelong education enhances their capacity to provide the best possible care to patients facing diverse medical conditions, irrespective of the ever-changing landscape of healthcare.

Chapter 15 underscores that CNAs are not merely caregivers but also knowledgeable healthcare professionals who occupy pivotal roles in managing a myriad of pathologies. By honing their understanding of pathology knowledge, expertly recognizing symptoms, fostering effective collaboration within the healthcare team, and dedicating themselves to lifelong learning, CNAs ensure they are well-prepared to offer empathetic, informed, and exceptional care to patients grappling with a wide spectrum of medical conditions. Their dedication to these principles is a testament to their unwavering commitment to the well-being and healthcare journeys of those under their care.

Chapter 16

CNA Continuing Education

Continuous learning and professional development are essential components of a successful career as a Certified Nursing Assistant (CNA). In Chapter 16 of "CNA for All," we explore the significance of ongoing education and growth in the field of healthcare. Real-life examples and detailed insights illustrate how CNAs can proactively engage in professional development to enhance their knowledge, skills, and career opportunities.

The Importance of Professional Development

Professional development is not only beneficial for CNAs themselves but also crucial for maintaining high-quality patient care. Staying updated with the latest healthcare advancements, regulations, and best practices ensures that CNAs provide the best possible care to their patients.

Imagine Sarah, a CNA in a hospital, who recognizes the importance of professional development. She regularly attends workshops and seminars to expand her knowledge and skills. By staying informed about new techniques in patient care and advancements in medical technology, Sarah can provide more effective care to her patients and stay competitive in her career.

Continuing Education Opportunities

CNAs have access to a variety of continuing education opportunities that can help them grow professionally. These include formal education programs, online courses, in-service training, and certifications in specialized areas of care.

In a long-term care facility, Mark, a CNA, takes advantage of continuing education opportunities offered by his employer. He pursues certification in geriatric care to enhance his skills in caring for elderly residents. This additional training not only benefits Mark's professional growth but also elevates the quality of care he provides to residents.

Staying Informed About Regulations

Healthcare regulations and guidelines are constantly evolving, and CNAs must stay informed about these changes to ensure they are providing care that complies with legal and ethical standards.

Emily, a CNA working in a rehabilitation center, understands the importance of staying updated with regulations. She regularly reviews updates in infection control guidelines and other healthcare regulations to ensure that her practices align with the latest recommendations. Emily's commitment to compliance not only reduces the risk of healthcare-associated infections but also demonstrates her dedication to patient safety.

Career Advancement Opportunities

Professional development also opens doors to career advancement for CNAs. With additional training, certifications, and experience, CNAs can pursue roles with more responsibilities and higher pay.

In a nursing home, Jessica, a CNA, aspires to advance her career. She completes a medication aide training program and obtains the necessary certification. With her newfound skills, Jessica takes on a medication administration role within the facility, which not only increases her earning potential but also allows her to contribute to residents' medication management.

Personal Growth and Fulfillment

Professional development is not just about career advancement; it also contributes to personal growth and job satisfaction. CNAs who actively engage in learning often find their work more fulfilling and rewarding.

Chapter 17

Effective Healthcare Collaboration

Effective communication and collaboration are the cornerstones of successful healthcare delivery. In Chapter 17 of "CNA for All," we explore the critical importance of communication skills and teamwork in the daily practice of Certified Nursing Assistants (CNAs). Real-life examples and detailed insights illustrate how CNAs foster effective communication and collaboration to enhance patient care and outcomes.

The Role of Effective Communication

Effective communication is fundamental in healthcare. CNAs must communicate clearly, compassionately, and efficiently with patients, families, and healthcare team members.

Consider Sarah, a CNA in a long-term care facility, caring for Mrs. Johnson, a resident with a complex medical history. Sarah engages in open and empathetic communication with Mrs. Johnson, ensuring she understands her care plan and preferences. Sarah also communicates changes in Mrs. Johnson's condition to the nursing team promptly. Her effective communication ensures that Mrs. Johnson receives personalized care that meets her needs.

Patient-Centered Care

Patient-centered care is a key concept in healthcare, emphasizing the importance of involving patients in their care decisions and respecting their values and preferences. CNAs play a pivotal role in delivering patient-centered care through effective communication.

In a hospital setting, Mark, a CNA, cares for Emily, a patient recovering from surgery. Mark actively engages Emily in discussions about her pain management, mobility goals, and discharge plans. He listens to her concerns and preferences, ensuring that her care aligns with her individual needs and values. Mark's patient-centered approach enhances Emily's sense of control and satisfaction with her care.

Interdisciplinary Collaboration

Collaboration is essential in healthcare, as CNAs work alongside nurses, physicians, therapists, and other healthcare professionals to provide comprehensive care. Effective collaboration requires clear communication and mutual respect.

Emily, a CNA in a rehabilitation center, collaborates with physical therapists to help a patient, Mr. Anderson, regain his mobility. She communicates regularly with the therapy team to provide insight into Mr. Anderson's progress and challenges. This collaboration ensures that Mr. Anderson receives coordinated care that accelerates his recovery.

Conflict Resolution

Conflict may arise in healthcare settings due to differing opinions or misunderstandings. CNAs must be skilled in conflict resolution to ensure that patient care is not compromised.

Imagine Jessica, a CNA in a long-term care facility, who encounters a disagreement with a colleague regarding a resident's care plan. Instead of allowing the conflict to escalate, Jessica initiates a constructive conversation with her colleague, seeking to understand their perspective and find common ground. Her effective conflict resolution skills facilitate a resolution that benefits the resident's well-being.

Cultural Sensitivity

Cultural competence is essential in communication, as healthcare professionals encounter patients from diverse backgrounds. CNAs must be sensitive to cultural differences and adapt their communication styles accordingly.

Chapter 18

Handling Challenging Behaviors and Conflict Resolution

Certified Nursing Assistants (CNAs) often encounter challenging behaviors in their roles while providing care to patients. In Chapter 18 of "CNA for All," we delve into the importance of understanding, managing, and effectively addressing challenging behaviors in healthcare settings. Real-life examples and detailed insights illustrate how CNAs can navigate these situations with professionalism and compassion.

Understanding Challenging Behaviors

Challenging behaviors in healthcare can encompass a range of actions, including aggression, agitation, resistance to care, or expressions of distress. CNAs must first seek to understand the underlying causes of these behaviors to provide appropriate care.

Imagine Sarah, a CNA in a dementia care unit, caring for a resident, Mr. Johnson, who frequently exhibits agitation and restlessness. Sarah recognizes that Mr. Johnson's behaviors may be a response to discomfort, fear, or unmet needs. She communicates with the nursing team to conduct a comprehensive assessment of Mr. Johnson's physical and emotional well-being. By understanding the root causes of his behaviors, Sarah can tailor her care approach to better meet his needs.

De-escalation Techniques

De-escalation techniques are crucial skills for CNAs when faced with challenging behaviors. These techniques involve calming strategies and communication approaches to help diffuse tense situations.

In a long-term care facility, Mark, a CNA, encounters a resident, Mrs. Davis, who becomes agitated during personal care routines. Mark utilizes de-escalation techniques, such as speaking in a calm and soothing tone, providing reassurance, and allowing Mrs. Davis to express her concerns. His compassionate approach helps Mrs. Davis feel more at ease and willing to cooperate with her care.

Collaboration with the Healthcare Team

Addressing challenging behaviors often requires collaboration with the healthcare team. CNAs should communicate effectively with nurses, therapists, and other professionals to develop strategies and interventions for managing these behaviors.

Emily, a CNA in a psychiatric unit, cares for a patient, David, who exhibits aggressive outbursts. Emily communicates David's behavior patterns to the nursing team and collaborates with the unit's psychiatrist and therapist. Together, they develop a behavior management plan that incorporates interventions like redirection, therapeutic activities, and medication adjustments. Emily's teamwork and communication skills are essential in addressing David's challenging behaviors effectively.

Conflict Resolution Skills

CNAs may also encounter conflicts with patients, families, or colleagues. Conflict resolution skills are vital for maintaining a positive work environment and ensuring that patient care is not compromised.

Jessica, a CNA in a nursing home, experiences a disagreement with a family member regarding the resident's care plan. She employs conflict resolution techniques, such as active listening, seeking common ground, and involving the nursing team in the discussion. Jessica's ability to resolve the conflict amicably ensures that the resident's best interests are upheld, and the family member feels heard and valued.

Chapter 19

Palliative and End-of-Life Care

Palliative and end-of-life care are specialized areas of healthcare that require unique skills, empathy, and sensitivity. In Chapter 19 of "CNA for All," we explore the essential role of Certified Nursing Assistants (CNAs) in providing palliative and end-of-life care to patients and their families. Real-life examples and detailed insights illustrate how CNAs offer comfort, dignity, and support during these profound moments.

Understanding Palliative and End-of-Life Care

Palliative care focuses on relieving pain and suffering in patients with serious illnesses, while end-of-life care provides support to individuals nearing the end of their lives. CNAs play a crucial role in both areas, ensuring that patients experience comfort and dignity during these sensitive times.

Consider Sarah, a CNA in a hospice facility, caring for a patient, Mr. Johnson, who has terminal cancer. Sarah understands that her role extends beyond physical care; it involves providing emotional support, active listening, and creating a peaceful environment. By embracing palliative and end-of-life care principles, Sarah helps Mr. Johnson and his family navigate this challenging journey.

Pain and Symptom Management

Effective pain and symptom management are vital components of palliative and end-of-life care. CNAs must work closely with the healthcare team to ensure that patients are as comfortable as possible.

In a hospital's palliative care unit, Mark, a CNA, provides care to Emily, a patient with advanced heart disease. Mark assists with administering pain medication and monitors Emily's comfort levels closely. He communicates any changes in her condition to the nursing team promptly. Mark's dedication to pain and symptom management helps alleviate Emily's suffering and ensures her comfort.

Emotional Support for Patients and Families

Palliative and end-of-life care often involve complex emotional and psychological needs. CNAs must be empathetic listeners and provide emotional support not only to patients but also to their families.

Imagine Emily, a CNA in a home care setting, caring for a terminally ill patient, Maria. Emily takes the time to sit with Maria and listen to her fears and concerns. She also offers support and guidance to Maria's family members, who are struggling with their loved one's impending passing. Emily's compassionate presence brings solace and reassurance to both Maria and her family during this difficult time.

Maintaining Dignity and Comfort

Preserving the dignity and comfort of patients is a fundamental principle of palliative and end-of-life care. CNAs must be attentive to patients' needs and preferences, helping them maintain their sense of identity and autonomy.

In a nursing home, Jessica, a CNA, cares for Mr. Thompson, a resident in the final stages of a terminal illness. Jessica ensures that Mr. Thompson's personal preferences and choices are respected, even as his care needs intensify. By upholding Mr. Thompson's dignity and comfort, Jessica helps him experience a peaceful and dignified end of life.

Chapter 19 underscores that CNAs are essential in providing palliative and end-of-life care that is compassionate and dignified. By understanding the principles of palliative care, effectively managing pain and symptoms, offering emotional support to patients and families, and preserving dignity and comfort, CNAs contribute significantly to the well-being and quality of life of individuals in their final moments, leaving a lasting impact on those they serve.

Chapter 20

Patient Safety in CNA Practice

Ensuring quality improvement and patient safety are paramount in healthcare, and Certified Nursing Assistants (CNAs) play a crucial role in these efforts. Chapter 20 of "CNA for All" explores the significance of continuously improving care and maintaining a safe environment for patients. Real-life examples and detailed insights illustrate how CNAs contribute to quality improvement and patient safety.

The Importance of Quality Improvement

Quality improvement in healthcare involves a systematic approach to enhancing the delivery of care, reducing errors, and improving patient outcomes. CNAs must actively participate in quality improvement initiatives to provide the best possible care.

Consider Sarah, a CNA in a long-term care facility, who notices that residents frequently experience falls in a specific hallway. Sarah raises this concern during staff meetings and collaborates with the nursing team to implement fall prevention strategies. Her proactive approach not only reduces fall rates but also enhances the overall quality of care provided in the facility.

Patient Safety

Patient safety is a fundamental principle in healthcare, and CNAs are responsible for ensuring that patients are protected from harm. This includes preventing accidents, infections, and medication errors.

In a hospital setting, Mark, a CNA, consistently adheres to patient safety protocols. He follows proper hand hygiene practices to prevent infections, checks patient identification before administering medications, and assists patients with mobility to reduce the risk of falls. Mark's dedication to patient safety safeguards the well-being of patients in his care.

Reporting and Documentation

Accurate reporting and documentation are essential aspects of quality improvement and patient safety. CNAs must communicate effectively with the healthcare team and document all relevant information regarding patient care.

Emily, a CNA in a rehabilitation center, encounters a patient, Mr. Anderson, who experiences a sudden change in his condition. Emily promptly reports the change to the nursing staff, providing detailed information about Mr. Anderson's vital signs and symptoms. Her timely and thorough reporting allows for rapid intervention, contributing to Mr. Anderson's improved outcome.

Continuous Education and Training

Staying updated with the latest healthcare practices through education and training is vital for CNAs to ensure patient safety and the delivery of high-quality care.

Imagine Jessica, a CNA in a long-term care facility, who regularly participates in training sessions on infection control and safe patient handling. Her commitment to continuous education not only enhances her knowledge and skills but also reduces the risk of healthcare-associated infections and patient injuries in the facility.

Participating in Quality Improvement Teams

Many healthcare facilities have quality improvement teams or committees that CNAs can join. These teams focus on identifying areas for improvement and implementing changes to enhance patient care and safety.

Chapter 21

Caring for Patients with Cognitive Impairments

Caring for patients with cognitive impairments presents unique challenges and requires specialized skills and understanding. In Chapter 21 of "CNA for All," we explore the essential role of Certified Nursing Assistants (CNAs) in providing compassionate and effective care to individuals with conditions such as dementia and Alzheimer's disease. Real-life examples and detailed insights illustrate how CNAs can meet the specific needs of these patients while upholding their dignity and quality of life.

Understanding Cognitive Impairments

Cognitive impairments, such as dementia and Alzheimer's disease, affect a person's memory, thinking, and decision-making abilities. CNAs must have a thorough understanding of these conditions to provide appropriate care.

Consider Sarah, a CNA in a memory care unit, caring for residents with various stages of dementia. Sarah has received specialized training in dementia care, enabling her to recognize the unique challenges residents face. She understands the importance of using clear and simple communication techniques to engage with residents and alleviate their distress.

Person-Centered Care

Person-centered care is the foundation of providing care to individuals with cognitive impairments. CNAs must tailor their care approaches to meet each patient's specific needs, preferences, and routines.

In a long-term care facility, Mark, a CNA, cares for Mr. Johnson, a resident with Alzheimer's disease. Mark takes the time to learn about Mr. Johnson's life history, hobbies, and interests. By incorporating this knowledge into his care routine, Mark engages Mr. Johnson in meaningful activities that promote a sense of purpose and well-being.

Effective Communication

Effective communication is crucial when caring for patients with cognitive impairments. CNAs must use clear and simple language, maintain eye contact, and employ non-verbal cues to convey information and provide reassurance.

Imagine Emily, a CNA in a home care setting, caring for a patient, Maria, who has dementia. Emily uses gentle and reassuring communication techniques to help Maria with daily activities. She patiently explains each step of the care process, reducing Maria's anxiety and ensuring her comfort.

Managing Behavioral Challenges

Patients with cognitive impairments may exhibit behavioral challenges, such as agitation, aggression, or wandering. CNAs must be equipped with strategies to manage and de-escalate these behaviors while preserving patient dignity.

In a nursing home, Jessica, a CNA, cares for residents with varying degrees of cognitive impairment. When a resident becomes agitated and refuses care, Jessica employs redirection techniques, offers comfort, and allows the resident to make choices when appropriate. Her compassionate approach minimizes behavioral challenges and promotes a calm and safe environment.

Supporting Families

Caring for patients with cognitive impairments often involves providing support and education to their families. CNAs can be a valuable resource for families, offering guidance and reassurance during challenging times.

Chapter 21 underscores that CNAs are pivotal in providing compassionate care to individuals with cognitive impairments. By understanding these conditions, embracing person-centered care, communicating effectively, managing behavioral challenges with dignity, and supporting patients' families, CNAs can enhance the quality of life for those living with cognitive impairments and create an environment of comfort and understanding.

Chapter 22

Cultural Competence in CNA Practice

Cultural competence is an essential aspect of providing high-quality and patient-centered care. In Chapter 22 of "CNA for All," we explore the significance of cultural competence in the practice of Certified Nursing Assistants (CNAs). Real-life examples and detailed insights illustrate how CNAs can effectively care for patients from diverse cultural backgrounds while respecting their values, beliefs, and traditions.

The Importance of Cultural Competence

Cultural competence involves the ability to understand, respect, and provide care that is sensitive to the cultural backgrounds and beliefs of patients. It is crucial for CNAs to recognize and embrace cultural diversity to deliver inclusive and respectful care.

Consider Sarah, a CNA in a multicultural healthcare facility, where she cares for patients from various cultural backgrounds. Sarah takes the time to learn about her patients' cultural traditions, dietary preferences, and communication styles. By incorporating cultural competence into her care, Sarah ensures that each patient feels valued and respected.

Effective Communication Across Cultures

Effective communication is at the core of cultural competence. CNAs must be skilled in adapting their communication styles to accommodate patients with diverse linguistic and cultural backgrounds.

In a hospital setting, Mark, a CNA, cares for a patient, Mrs. Gomez, who primarily speaks Spanish. Although Mark is not fluent in Spanish, he uses simple and clear language, employs visual aids, and seeks the assistance of a medical interpreter when necessary. His efforts in effective cross-cultural communication ensure that Mrs. Gomez receives accurate information and feels heard and understood.

Respecting Cultural Beliefs and Practices

Respecting cultural beliefs and practices is a fundamental principle of cultural competence. CNAs must honor patients' customs, traditions, and spiritual beliefs while providing care.

Imagine Emily, a CNA in a hospice care facility, caring for a patient, Mr. Kim, from a culture that places a strong emphasis on family decision-making. Emily ensures that Mr. Kim's family is actively involved in his care decisions and provides space for traditional rituals and ceremonies to be conducted. Her respect for Mr. Kim's cultural values and practices supports his emotional well-being.

Addressing Health Disparities

Cultural competence is also linked to addressing health disparities. CNAs play a crucial role in advocating for equitable care and identifying disparities that may exist within healthcare systems.

In a long-term care facility, Jessica, a CNA, notices that residents from certain cultural backgrounds are less likely to engage in social activities due to language barriers. She communicates this concern to the facility's management, advocating for increased access to interpreters and culturally tailored activities. Jessica's advocacy helps bridge gaps in care and improve the overall well-being of residents from diverse cultural backgrounds.

Continuous Cultural Education

Cultural competence is an ongoing journey, and CNAs must continually educate themselves about different cultures and remain open to learning from their patients.

Chapter 23

Ethical Dilemmas in CNA Practice

Certified Nursing Assistants (CNAs) often encounter complex ethical dilemmas while providing care to patients. In Chapter 23 of "CNA for All," we delve into the challenging situations that CNAs may face and explore the ethical principles and decision-making processes that guide their actions. Real-life examples and detailed insights illustrate how CNAs navigate these dilemmas with compassion and professionalism.

The Nature of Ethical Dilemmas

Ethical dilemmas in healthcare are situations where CNAs are confronted with conflicting values, principles, or obligations. These dilemmas can arise from issues related to patient autonomy, privacy, truth-telling, and allocation of resources.

Consider Sarah, a CNA in a long-term care facility, who is asked by a family member to withhold information from an elderly resident about a terminal diagnosis. This request places Sarah in an ethical dilemma as she must balance the resident's right to know about their condition with the family's desire to protect them from distressing news.

Patient Autonomy and Informed Consent

Patient autonomy is a fundamental ethical principle in healthcare, emphasizing a patient's right to make decisions about their own care. CNAs must respect this autonomy and ensure that patients are informed and can provide informed consent for their treatments.

In a hospital setting, Mark, a CNA, cares for a patient, Emily, who is considering a surgical procedure. Mark ensures that Emily receives all the necessary information about the procedure, its risks, and benefits. He encourages her to ask questions and consult with the medical team. By supporting Emily's informed decision-making, Mark upholds the principle of patient autonomy.

Confidentiality and Privacy

Maintaining patient confidentiality and privacy is another ethical obligation for CNAs. They must safeguard patients' personal and medical information to protect their dignity and rights.

Imagine Emily, a CNA in a rehabilitation center, who overhears a colleague discussing a patient's medical history in a public area. Emily promptly reminds her colleague about the importance of respecting patient confidentiality and reporting such breaches to the appropriate authorities. Her commitment to confidentiality preserves patients' trust and privacy.

End-of-Life Dilemmas

End-of-life care can present complex ethical dilemmas, especially when patients have advanced directives or family members with differing views on treatment options.

In a nursing home, Jessica, a CNA, cares for a resident who has a do-not-resuscitate (DNR) order in place. When a family member insists on calling 911 during a medical emergency, Jessica must navigate the ethical dilemma of honoring the resident's wishes while respecting the family's concerns. She engages in open and compassionate communication with the family to find a solution that aligns with the resident's preferences.

Ethical Decision-Making

Ethical decision-making involves a thoughtful process where CNAs weigh the moral principles at stake, consult with colleagues and healthcare professionals, and seek guidance from ethical codes and policies.

Chapter 24

Self-Care and Burnout Prevention for CNAs

Self-care is a vital aspect of maintaining physical and emotional well-being for Certified Nursing Assistants (CNAs). In Chapter 24 of "CNA for All," we explore the importance of self-care and strategies to prevent burnout in the demanding field of healthcare. Real-life examples and detailed insights illustrate how CNAs can prioritize their own health while providing quality care to patients.

Understanding the Demands of the CNA Role

Working as a CNA can be physically and emotionally demanding. CNAs are often responsible for providing direct patient care, assisting with activities of daily living, and supporting patients in challenging situations. This can lead to high levels of stress and burnout if self-care is neglected.

Consider Sarah, a CNA in a busy hospital, who works long shifts and frequently encounters emotionally charged situations. Without proper self-care, Sarah could find herself physically exhausted and emotionally drained, affecting her ability to provide quality care.

The Importance of Self-Care

Self-care is not a luxury; it is a necessity for CNAs. Taking care of oneself is essential for maintaining physical and mental health, sustaining energy levels, and providing the best care possible to patients.

In a long-term care facility, Mark, a CNA, recognizes the importance of self-care. He ensures he gets adequate rest between shifts, engages in regular exercise, and practices mindfulness to manage stress. By prioritizing his own well-being, Mark is better equipped to provide compassionate care to his residents.

Recognizing the Signs of Burnout

Burnout is a state of emotional, physical, and mental exhaustion that results from prolonged stress and overwork. CNAs must be aware of the signs of burnout, which may include feelings of cynicism, decreased job satisfaction, and physical symptoms like fatigue and sleep disturbances.

Imagine Emily, a CNA in a rehabilitation center, who notices that she is becoming increasingly irritable and has difficulty concentrating. She recognizes these as signs of burnout and takes action to address her well-being before it escalates.

Self-Care Strategies

Effective self-care strategies for CNAs encompass physical, emotional, and mental well-being. CNAs can consider the following approaches:

1. **Balanced Diet**: Consuming a nutritious diet supports energy levels and overall health.

2. **Physical Activity**: Regular exercise helps manage stress and boost mood.

3. **Restorative Sleep**: Quality sleep is essential for rejuvenating the body and mind.

4. **Mindfulness and Relaxation**: Practicing relaxation techniques and mindfulness can reduce stress.

5. **Seeking Support**: CNAs should not hesitate to seek emotional support from friends, family, or mental health professionals.

6. **Setting Boundaries**: Establishing clear boundaries between work and personal life is crucial to prevent burnout.

7. **Time Management**: Efficiently managing time and prioritizing tasks can reduce stress and improve work-life balance.

Chapter 25

Adapting to Technological Advancements in CNA Practice

The healthcare industry has seen significant technological advancements in recent years, transforming the way care is provided and documented. In Chapter 25 of "CNA for All," we explore the integration of technology into the role of Certified Nursing Assistants (CNAs). Real-life examples and detailed insights illustrate how CNAs can adapt to and leverage these advancements to enhance patient care and their own efficiency.

The Evolution of Healthcare Technology

Advances in healthcare technology have brought about changes in various aspects of patient care, from electronic health records (EHRs) to telehealth services. CNAs are increasingly exposed to these technological tools, which can streamline workflows and improve the quality of care.

Consider Sarah, a CNA in a hospital, who now uses electronic tablets to access patient records, input vital signs, and communicate with the nursing team. The integration of technology has made Sarah's documentation more efficient and accessible, allowing her to focus more on direct patient care.

Utilizing Electronic Health Records (EHRs)

EHRs have become a standard in healthcare, allowing for the digital storage and retrieval of patient information. CNAs must become proficient in using EHR systems to access patient records, document care, and communicate with the healthcare team.

In a long-term care facility, Mark, a CNA, uses EHRs to review care plans, document patient progress, and report any changes in residents' conditions. This electronic documentation ensures that important information is readily available to the entire care team, promoting coordinated and informed care.

Telehealth and Remote Monitoring

Telehealth services and remote monitoring have expanded access to healthcare for many patients, especially those in remote areas. CNAs may find themselves involved in facilitating telehealth appointments and assisting with remote patient monitoring.

Emily, a CNA in a home care setting, helps patients connect with their healthcare providers through telehealth appointments. She ensures that patients understand how to use the technology and assists with setting up virtual visits. This technology allows patients to receive timely care while remaining in the comfort of their homes.

Ensuring Data Security and Privacy

As CNAs use technology to access and input patient information, they must be vigilant in maintaining data security and patient privacy. Adhering to HIPAA regulations and facility policies is paramount to protect patient information.

In a hospital's computerized charting system, Jessica, a CNA, follows strict protocols to ensure patient data remains confidential. She uses secure login credentials, avoids discussing patient information in public areas, and reports any potential security breaches promptly.

Continuous Learning and Adaptation

Technology in healthcare is continuously evolving, and CNAs must be open to learning and adapting to new tools and systems. Staying updated with the latest technological advancements ensures that CNAs remain proficient in their roles.

Chapter 25 underscores that technology is becoming increasingly integrated into the practice of CNAs. By embracing EHRs, facilitating telehealth services, ensuring data security and privacy, and committing to continuous learning and adaptation, CNAs can leverage technology to enhance patient care, improve documentation accuracy, and streamline communication.

Chapter 26

Disaster Preparedness and Response in CNA Practice

Disasters, whether natural or man-made, can strike unexpectedly and have a profound impact on healthcare settings. In Chapter 26 of "CNA for All," we explore the critical role of Certified Nursing Assistants (CNAs) in disaster preparedness and response. Real-life examples and detailed insights illustrate how CNAs can contribute to the safety and well-being of patients and themselves during emergency situations.

The Importance of Disaster Preparedness

Disaster preparedness is a crucial component of healthcare. CNAs must be proactive in preparing for potential disasters, as their role places them on the front lines of patient care during emergencies.

Consider Sarah, a CNA in a healthcare facility located in an area prone to hurricanes. Sarah and her colleagues participate in regular disaster drills and training sessions to ensure they are well-prepared to respond effectively when a disaster strikes.

Roles and Responsibilities During Disasters

CNAs have specific roles and responsibilities during disasters, which may include evacuating patients, assisting with triage, providing basic first aid, and maintaining clear communication with the healthcare team.

In a hospital facing a sudden power outage, Mark, a CNA, collaborates with nurses and other staff to safely transfer patients to areas with emergency power. Mark's knowledge of patient needs and his ability to work efficiently under pressure contribute to a smooth response during the crisis.

Patient Evacuation and Sheltering

During disasters, patient evacuation may become necessary to ensure their safety. CNAs may be involved in transporting patients to designated shelters or assisting with their evacuation.

Emily, a CNA in a nursing home, helps evacuate residents when flooding threatens the facility. She ensures that residents are safely transferred to buses and shelters while prioritizing their comfort and well-being during the process.

Psychological Support

Disasters can be traumatic experiences for patients and their families. CNAs must provide emotional support, reassurance, and clear communication to alleviate anxiety and stress.

Jessica, a CNA in an assisted living facility, provides comfort to residents and their families during a wildfire evacuation. Her calming presence and empathetic communication help ease residents' fears and foster a sense of security.

Personal Preparedness

In addition to their professional responsibilities, CNAs should also prioritize personal disaster preparedness. This includes having an emergency kit, knowing evacuation routes, and having a plan in place for their own families.

Chapter 26 emphasizes that CNAs are vital in disaster preparedness and response. By actively participating in disaster drills, understanding their roles and responsibilities, facilitating patient evacuation and sheltering, offering psychological support, and ensuring personal preparedness, CNAs play a crucial role in safeguarding the well-being of patients and contributing to the overall resilience of healthcare facilities during emergencies.

Chapter 27

Interdisciplinary Collaboration in CNA Practice

Interdisciplinary collaboration is a cornerstone of effective healthcare delivery, and Certified Nursing Assistants (CNAs) play a pivotal role in this collaborative effort. In Chapter 27 of "CNA for All," we explore the significance of working closely with other healthcare professionals to provide comprehensive and patient-centered care. Real-life examples and detailed insights illustrate how CNAs can contribute to successful interdisciplinary collaboration.

The Importance of Interdisciplinary Collaboration

Healthcare is a complex field that often requires the expertise of various professionals, including nurses, physicians, therapists, social workers, and CNAs. Effective interdisciplinary collaboration ensures that each team member's unique skills and knowledge are leveraged to provide the best care possible.

Consider Sarah, a CNA in a rehabilitation center, where patients receive care from a diverse team of professionals. Sarah understands that successful rehabilitation outcomes rely on the collective efforts of the interdisciplinary team, including therapists, nurses, and herself.

Clear Communication and Information Sharing

Clear communication is essential in interdisciplinary collaboration. CNAs must be adept at sharing relevant information about patient conditions, needs, and changes in status with other team members.

In a long-term care facility, Mark, a CNA, communicates regularly with the nursing team about residents' vital signs and any changes in their conditions. Mark's detailed and timely reports allow nurses to make informed decisions about resident care, ensuring that any issues are addressed promptly.

Collaboration in Care Planning

Interdisciplinary collaboration is particularly crucial in the development and implementation of individualized care plans. CNAs contribute their observations and insights about patients to ensure that care plans are comprehensive and responsive to patients' needs.

Emily, a CNA in a home care setting, actively participates in care planning meetings with a team of healthcare professionals, including a nurse, therapist, and social worker. Emily's input regarding the patient's daily routines and preferences helps create a care plan that respects the patient's individuality and maximizes their well-being.

Respecting Each Team Member's Expertise

Effective collaboration requires recognizing and respecting each team member's expertise. CNAs should appreciate the unique contributions of nurses, therapists, and other professionals while also valuing their own role in patient care.

Jessica, a CNA in a hospital, demonstrates this respect by seeking guidance from nurses and therapists when needed while also confidently providing essential daily care to patients. Her ability to collaborate seamlessly with the interdisciplinary team ensures that patients receive comprehensive and coordinated care.

Conflict Resolution and Team Dynamics

In healthcare, disagreements and conflicts can arise among team members due to differences in opinions or approaches. CNAs should be skilled in conflict resolution and be proactive in fostering positive team dynamics.

Chapter 27 underscores that CNAs are integral members of the interdisciplinary healthcare team. By emphasizing clear communication and information sharing, active participation in care planning, respecting each team member's expertise, and addressing conflict resolution and team dynamics, CNAs contribute to the overall success of patient care.

Chapter 28

Ethical Considerations in End-of-Life Care

End-of-life care is a profoundly sensitive and complex aspect of healthcare, and Certified Nursing Assistants (CNAs) play a crucial role in ensuring that patients at the end of their lives receive compassionate and dignified care. In Chapter 28 of "CNA for All," we explore the ethical considerations that guide CNAs in providing end-of-life care. Real-life examples and detailed insights illustrate how CNAs navigate these complex situations with empathy and professionalism.

The Ethical Dimensions of End-of-Life Care

End-of-life care involves a range of ethical considerations, including respecting patient autonomy, maintaining dignity, preserving comfort, and supporting families during difficult times. CNAs must be attuned to these ethical principles to provide the best care possible.

Consider Sarah, a CNA in a hospice facility, who cares for a patient, Mr. Johnson, in the final stages of a terminal illness. Sarah understands the importance of upholding Mr. Johnson's autonomy by involving him in care decisions and respecting his choices about pain management and treatment options.

Preserving Dignity and Comfort

Preserving the dignity and comfort of patients at the end of life is a fundamental ethical principle. CNAs must be attentive to patients' physical, emotional, and psychological needs to ensure they experience a peaceful and dignified transition.

In a nursing home, Mark, a CNA, cares for Ms. Thompson, a resident in her final days. Mark ensures that Ms. Thompson's personal preferences and choices are respected, even as her care needs intensify. By upholding Ms. Thompson's dignity and comfort, Mark helps her experience a dignified end of life.

Effective Communication and Emotional Support

Effective communication is essential in end-of-life care, as patients and their families may have difficult decisions to make and complex emotions to navigate. CNAs must provide emotional support, active listening, and empathetic presence to patients and their loved ones.

Imagine Emily, a CNA in a home care setting, caring for a terminally ill patient, Maria. Emily takes the time to sit with Maria and listen to her fears and concerns. She also offers support and guidance to Maria's family members, who are struggling with their loved one's impending passing. Emily's compassionate presence brings solace and reassurance to both Maria and her family during this difficult time.

Ethical Decision-Making at the End of Life

Ethical decision-making is particularly challenging in end-of-life care, where complex choices about treatments, pain management, and resuscitation may arise. CNAs must collaborate with the healthcare team, patients, and families to make decisions that align with the patient's values and preferences.

In a hospital's palliative care unit, Jessica, a CNA, is part of a care team discussing the appropriate level of interventions for a patient with advanced illness. Jessica advocates for a care plan that focuses on comfort and quality of life, aligning with the patient's wishes. Her input contributes to a more ethically sound and patient-centered approach.

Chapter 29

Advocacy and Patient Rights in CNA Practice

Advocacy is an essential component of nursing care, and Certified Nursing Assistants (CNAs) often serve as strong advocates for their patients. In Chapter 29 of "CNA for All," we delve into the critical role of CNAs in advocating for patient rights, safety, and well-being. Real-life examples and detailed insights illustrate how CNAs can effectively advocate for their patients in a healthcare setting.

Understanding the Role of Advocacy

Advocacy in healthcare involves speaking up on behalf of patients to ensure their rights and best interests are protected. CNAs must understand their role as advocates and be prepared to act in the best interest of their patients.

Consider Sarah, a CNA in a long-term care facility, who notices that a resident's pain medication is consistently late, leading to unnecessary discomfort. Sarah advocates for the resident by raising this issue with the nursing team and suggesting adjustments to the medication administration schedule.

Promoting Patient Rights

Patient rights encompass a wide range of principles, including the right to informed consent, privacy, dignity, and respectful treatment. CNAs are responsible for upholding and promoting these rights in their interactions with patients.

In a hospital, Mark, a CNA, ensures that patients are informed about their care and treatment options. He takes the time to explain procedures, answer questions, and seek informed consent. Mark's commitment to promoting patient rights helps patients feel respected and empowered in their healthcare decisions.

Ensuring Safe and Quality Care

Advocacy also extends to ensuring that patients receive safe and quality care. CNAs should be vigilant in identifying potential safety concerns, such as medication errors, fall risks, or inadequate infection control measures.

Emily, a CNA in a rehabilitation center, observes that some patients are not receiving proper assistance with mobility, putting them at risk of falls. Emily advocates for improved safety measures, including additional staff training and better equipment. Her advocacy helps prevent injuries and enhance the quality of care.

Effective Communication and Collaboration

Advocacy often involves effective communication and collaboration with the healthcare team. CNAs must be able to express their concerns, share observations, and work together with nurses, physicians, and other professionals to address issues affecting patient care.

Imagine Jessica, a CNA in a long-term care facility, who notices that a resident's wound is not healing as expected. She communicates her concerns to the nursing staff, collaborates with the wound care team, and advocates for a reevaluation of the treatment plan. Jessica's advocacy leads to better wound management and improved patient outcomes.

Supporting Vulnerable Populations

CNAs may also find themselves advocating for vulnerable populations, such as residents in long-term care facilities or patients with limited English proficiency. Ensuring that these individuals receive equal access to care and that their voices are heard is a critical aspect of advocacy.

Chapter 30

Professional Growth and Development for CNAs

The journey of a Certified Nursing Assistant (CNA) doesn't end with certification. In Chapter 30 of "CNA for All," we explore the importance of ongoing professional growth and development for CNAs. Real-life examples and detailed insights illustrate how CNAs can continue to enhance their skills, knowledge, and careers throughout their healthcare journey.

The Continual Learning Process

Healthcare is a dynamic field, with new discoveries, technologies, and best practices emerging regularly. CNAs must recognize that their role requires continual learning and growth to provide the best care possible.

Consider Sarah, a CNA in a skilled nursing facility, who takes advantage of opportunities for continuing education. She attends workshops, webinars, and courses to stay updated on the latest caregiving techniques and regulations. Sarah's commitment to learning ensures that she can adapt to changes in the healthcare environment.

Certifications and Specializations

CNAs can pursue additional certifications and specializations to expand their knowledge and career opportunities. These certifications can be in areas such as wound care, dementia care, or medication administration, allowing CNAs to take on more specialized roles.

In a hospital, Mark, a CNA, decides to pursue a certification in phlebotomy to assist with blood draws and specimen collection. This additional certification not only enhances Mark's skills but also opens up new avenues for him within the healthcare field.

Mentorship and Collaboration

Mentorship and collaboration with experienced healthcare professionals, including nurses and therapists, can significantly contribute to a CNA's growth and development. Learning from the expertise of others can offer valuable insights and enhance one's caregiving abilities.

Emily, a CNA in a home care setting, seeks mentorship from a seasoned nurse who guides complex care procedures and problem-solving. Emily's collaboration with the nurse enriches her skills and boosts her confidence in providing high-quality care.

Leadership and Career Advancement

CNAs with a passion for leadership and advancement can explore opportunities to become certified nursing assistants in leadership or management roles. These roles may involve supervisory responsibilities and require strong organizational and leadership skills.

Jessica, a CNA in a long-term care facility, aspires to take on a leadership role. She pursues additional training and certifications that qualify her for a charge nurse position. Jessica's dedication to professional growth allows her to make a broader impact on patient care.

Professional Associations and Networking

Joining professional associations and networking with fellow CNAs and healthcare professionals can provide valuable resources and support for career development. These associations offer access to conferences, publications, and networking events that can enhance a CNA's knowledge and career prospects.

Chapter 30 underscores that professional growth and development are ongoing processes for CNAs. By embracing continual learning, pursuing certifications and specializations, seeking mentorship and collaboration, considering leadership and career advancement, and participating in professional associations and networking.

Chapter 31

List of Questions and Answers (1)

1. What does CNA stand for?

    - Certified Nursing Assistant

2. What are the primary responsibilities of a CNA?

    - Assisting patients with daily activities, taking vital signs, and providing basic medical care under the supervision of a nurse.

3. What is the role of a CNA in infection control?

    - Following proper hand hygiene, wearing personal protective equipment, and maintaining a clean environment.

4. How often should you change gloves when providing care to a patient?

    - Whenever they become soiled, torn, or after completing a specific task with one patient.

5. What is the purpose of taking a patient's vital signs?

    - To monitor their overall health and detect any abnormalities.

6. What are the four vital signs?

    - Temperature, pulse, respiration rate, and blood pressure.

7. How do you measure a patient's temperature?

    - Using a thermometer orally, rectally, or axillary (under the armpit).

8. What is a normal body temperature in Fahrenheit?

- 98.6°F (37°C)

9. Define pulse rate.

- The number of times the heart beats per minute.

10. Where is the radial pulse located?

- On the inside of the wrist, at the base of the thumb.

11. What is a normal resting heart rate for adults?

- 60-100 beats per minute.

12. What is respiration rate?

- The number of breaths a person takes per minute.

13. How should you count a patient's respirations without them noticing?

- By observing their chest rise and fall while appearing to take their pulse.

14. What is blood pressure, and how is it measured?

- Blood pressure is the force of blood against the walls of the arteries. It is measured using a sphygmomanometer and a stethoscope.

15. What is systolic blood pressure?

- The higher number in a blood pressure reading, representing the pressure when the heart contracts.

16. What is diastolic blood pressure?

- The lower number in a blood pressure reading, representing the pressure when the heart is at rest between beats.

73

17. What is the normal range for systolic blood pressure in adults?

    - 90-120 mm Hg

18. What is the normal range for diastolic blood pressure in adults?

    - 60-80 mm Hg

19. How do you properly transfer a patient from a bed to a wheelchair?

    - Use a transfer belt and assist the patient in a controlled manner.

20. When should you use a gait belt?

    - When assisting patients with walking or transferring.

21. What is the purpose of range of motion (ROM) exercises?

    - To maintain and improve joint mobility and prevent stiffness.

22. Describe passive range of motion exercises.

    - The caregiver moves the patient's joints through their full range of motion without the patient's assistance.

23. What is the purpose of documenting patient care?

    - To provide an accurate record of the patient's condition, care provided, and any changes in their health.

24. How often should you turn a bedridden patient to prevent pressure ulcers?

    - Every 2 hours.

25. What is the Heimlich maneuver, and when is it used?

- It is a procedure used to clear a blocked airway in a conscious choking adult or child.

26. What is the recovery position, and when should it be used?

- It is a safe position for an unconscious person, allowing for proper airway management. It should be used when the person is breathing but unresponsive.

27. What is the ABCD approach in CPR?

- Airway, Breathing, Circulation, and Defibrillation.

28. What should you do if a patient's breathing and pulse are absent?

- Begin CPR immediately.

29. How deep should chest compressions be during CPR for adults?

- At least 2 inches (5 cm).

30. What is the ratio of chest compressions to rescue breaths during CPR for adults?

- 30 compressions to 2 rescue breaths.

31. How do you provide CPR for infants?

- Using two fingers for chest compressions and covering the infant's mouth and nose for rescue breaths.

32. What is the purpose of a Code Blue in a healthcare facility?

- To respond to a cardiac or respiratory emergency.

33. What is the purpose of a Code Pink in a healthcare facility?

- To respond to a pediatric emergency.

34. Describe proper handwashing technique.

- Wet hands, apply soap, scrub for at least 20 seconds, rinse thoroughly, and dry with a clean towel.

35. What is the Chain of Infection, and how can it be broken?

- It is a series of events that allows infections to be transmitted. It can be broken by practicing good hand hygiene, using personal protective equipment, and following infection control protocols.

36. What is the role of a CNA in assisting with medication administration?

- CNAs are not typically allowed to administer medications but can remind patients to take their prescribed medications and report any concerns to a nurse.

37. What is a catheter, and why might a patient need one?

- A catheter is a tube inserted into the body to drain urine from the bladder. A patient might need one if they have difficulty urinating.

38. How often should you provide oral care for a patient with dentures?

- At least twice a day, and after meals.

39. What is the purpose of the Heel-Elbow Protectors (HEPs)?

- To prevent pressure ulcers on the heels and elbows of bedridden patients.

40. How can you promote independence and dignity in patients?

- Encourage them to perform tasks they are capable of, respect their choices, and maintain their privacy.

41. What is the difference between a sign and a symptom?

- A sign is an objective, observable indication of a medical condition, while a symptom is a subjective complaint reported by the patient.

42. What is the purpose of a bedpan, and how should it be positioned under a patient?

- A bedpan is used for patients who cannot get out of bed to use the toilet. It should be positioned with the wider end at the patient's buttocks.

43. How do you provide perineal care for a patient?

- Gently clean the genital and anal areas using a washcloth, soap, and water.

44. What is the proper way to assist a patient with dressing?

- Allow the patient to do as much as they can independently, assist with difficult tasks, and always respect their privacy.

45. What is the Braden Scale used for?

- To assess a patient's risk for developing pressure ulcers.

46. Describe the stages of pressure ulcers.

- Stage 1: Non-blanchable redness

- Stage 2: Partial-thickness skin loss

- Stage 3: Full-thickness skin loss

- Stage 4: Full-thickness skin and tissue loss

- Unstageable: Full-thickness loss with unknown depth

47. How should you handle a patient who is agitated or aggressive?

- Stay calm, use verbal de-escalation techniques, and call for assistance if necessary.

48. What is a urinary catheter, and why might it be used?

- A urinary catheter is a tube inserted into the bladder to drain urine. It might be used for patients with urinary retention, incontinence, or during surgery.

49. What is the purpose of a Foley catheter?

- To continuously drain urine from the bladder into a collection bag.

50. How often should you empty a urinary drainage bag?

- When it is half-full or as per facility policy.

51. How can you maintain a patient's dignity when assisting with toileting or hygiene?

- Close curtains, provide privacy, and communicate respectfully.

52. What is a Hoyer lift, and when is it used?

- A Hoyer lift is a device used to transfer immobile or heavy patients safely.

53. What is the primary goal of post-mortem care?

- To maintain the patient's dignity and prepare the body for viewing by family or funeral home personnel.

54. What is the purpose of an advanced directive?

- To specify a patient's healthcare wishes in advance in case they become unable to communicate or make decisions.

55. What is the difference between a living will and a durable power of attorney for healthcare?

- A living will outlines specific medical treatments a patient wants or doesn't want, while a durable power of attorney designates a person to make healthcare decisions on the patient's behalf.

56. What is the purpose of a bladder training program?

- To help patients regain control over their bladder and reduce urinary incontinence.

57. How can you assist a patient with a hearing impairment?

- Speak clearly and face the patient, use gestures or writing as needed, and provide hearing aids if applicable.

58. What is a bed sore, and what are the risk factors for developing one?

- A bed sore is a pressure ulcer that develops due to prolonged pressure on the skin. Risk factors include immobility, poor nutrition, moisture, and friction.

59. What is the purpose of a sitz bath, and when is it used?

- A sitz bath is used to provide relief for patients with perineal discomfort or inflammation.

60. How can you help prevent the development of pneumonia in bedridden patients?

- Encourage deep breathing and coughing exercises, and maintain proper positioning.

61. What is the purpose of a Foley catheter securement device?

- To prevent accidental dislodgement or pulling of the catheter.

62. Describe the proper way to provide oral care for an unconscious patient.

- Be gentle and use a foam swab or toothbrush with water or oral hygiene solution to clean the mouth.

63. What is the Glasgow Coma Scale (GCS), and how is it used?

- It is a neurological assessment tool used to evaluate a patient's level of consciousness based on eye, verbal, and motor responses.

64. How can you assist a patient with a visual impairment?

- Use verbal cues, identify yourself, and offer your arm for guidance when walking.

65. What is a code of ethics, and why is it important in healthcare?

- A code of ethics is a set of moral principles that guide the behavior and decision-making of healthcare professionals. It is important for maintaining trust and providing ethical care.

66. How can you help a patient with dysphagia (difficulty swallowing)?

- Follow the prescribed diet and ensure food and liquids are at the appropriate consistency.

67. What is the purpose of a tracheostomy tube?

- To provide a clear airway for patients who have difficulty breathing through the nose or mouth.

68. How often should you reposition a patient who is immobile in bed?

- At least every 2 hours.

69. What is the purpose of a fracture bedpan?

    - To assist patients with lower extremity fractures in positioning for toileting.

70. How can you help a patient with Alzheimer's or dementia feel more comfortable and secure?

    - Maintain a consistent routine, use reassuring communication, and create a familiar and safe environment.

71. Describe the proper technique for changing linens on an occupied bed.

    - Roll the patient to one side while changing the linens on the other side, then roll them to the opposite side to complete the bed change.

72. What is the role of a CNA in preventing falls in a healthcare setting?

    - Ensuring a safe environment, using bed and chair alarms when necessary, and assisting with mobility.

73. How can you assist a patient with diabetes in managing their condition?

    - Encourage regular blood glucose monitoring, help with insulin administration if needed, and promote a balanced diet.

74. What is a DNR (Do Not Resuscitate) order, and how should it be handled?

    - A DNR order specifies that a patient does not want life-saving measures in the event of cardiac or respiratory arrest. It should be respected, and the healthcare team should be informed.

75. What is the purpose of the Medical Power of Attorney (MPOA)?

- To designate a person to make medical decisions on behalf of a patient who is unable to make them.

76. How do you assist a patient with a urinary catheter in maintaining hygiene?

- Keep the catheter and surrounding area clean and dry, and ensure proper positioning of the drainage bag.

77. How can you help a patient who is experiencing shortness of breath?

- Assist with prescribed oxygen therapy, maintain proper positioning, and encourage deep breathing exercises.

78. What is the role of a CNA during the admission process for a new patient?

- Greeting and orienting the patient to their room, assisting with initial assessments, and providing emotional support.

79. How can you assist a patient with a mobility impairment?

- Use assistive devices such as wheelchairs or walkers, and follow proper transfer techniques.

80. What is the purpose of a feeding tube, and how should you care for it?

- A feeding tube provides nutrition for patients who cannot swallow. Care includes flushing with water, monitoring for complications, and proper positioning.

81. What is the purpose of a call light system in healthcare facilities?

- To allow patients to request assistance from the nursing staff.

82. How should you handle a situation where a patient refuses care?

Chapter 32

List of Questions and Answers (2)

1. What is the role of a Certified Nursing Assistant (CNA)?

    • CNAs provide basic patient care under the supervision of
    registered nurses (RNs) and doctors.

2. How can CNAs maintain patient confidentiality?

    • By not discussing patient information with unauthorized
    individuals and ensuring patient records are secure.

3. What is the first step in taking a patient's vital signs?

    • Checking their temperature.

4. What is a normal body temperature range for adults?

    • 97.8°F to 99.1°F (36.5°C to 37.3°C).

5. What is the purpose of measuring a patient's blood pressure?

    • To monitor their cardiovascular health and detect
    abnormalities.

6. What is a normal blood pressure reading for adults?

    • 120/80 mm Hg.

7. How often should a patient's position be changed to prevent bedsores?

    • Every 2 hours.

8. What is the purpose of providing oral hygiene for patients?

- To prevent dental issues, maintain oral health, and promote comfort.

9. How should a CNA assist a patient with feeding who has difficulty swallowing?

   - Offer small, manageable bites, and ensure the patient sits upright.

10. What should a CNA do if a patient refuses to eat?

    - Document the refusal and report it to the nurse.

11. How should a CNA assist a patient with toileting needs?

    - Provide privacy, assist with clothing, and help them to and from the toilet.

12. What is the purpose of measuring urinary output?

    - To monitor kidney function and hydration status.

13. How should a CNA assist a patient with a bedpan or urinal?

    - Ensure proper positioning, privacy, and hygiene.

14. What is the purpose of range-of-motion (ROM) exercises for patients?

    - To maintain joint mobility and prevent muscle atrophy.

15. How should a CNA communicate with patients who have dementia?

    - Use clear and simple language, maintain eye contact, and be patient.

16. What is the purpose of using restraints on patients?

- Restraints should be used as a last resort to prevent harm to the patient or others.

17. How can a CNA help prevent falls in a healthcare setting?

- By ensuring a safe environment, using bed alarms, and providing assistance when needed.

18. What is the role of a CNA during a code blue emergency?

- To assist the healthcare team by performing CPR, providing equipment, and documenting.

19. How can CNAs maintain infection control in their daily tasks?

- By proper handwashing, using personal protective equipment, and following isolation protocols.

20. What is the purpose of documenting patient care?

- To maintain accurate records of the patient's condition, treatments, and progress.

21. How should a CNA respond to a patient in pain?

- Report it to the nurse, provide comfort measures, and administer pain medication as ordered.

22. What is the CNA's responsibility during end-of-life care?

- To provide emotional support, maintain comfort, and respect the patient's wishes.

23. How can CNAs assist patients with mobility issues?

- Use assistive devices like walkers or wheelchairs and help with transfers.

24. What are pressure ulcers, and how can they be prevented?

- Pressure ulcers are skin injuries caused by prolonged pressure; prevention includes repositioning and proper skincare.

25. How should a CNA handle a patient with a communicable disease?

- Follow infection control procedures and use appropriate precautions.

26. What is the purpose of a urinary catheter, and how is it maintained?

- To drain urine when a patient cannot do so independently; it should be kept clean and sterile.

27. How should a CNA handle a patient experiencing a seizure?

- Protect the patient from harm, move objects out of the way, and stay with them until the seizure ends.

28. How can CNAs assist patients with mental health issues?

- Provide emotional support, engage in therapeutic communication, and report any concerning behaviors.

29. What is the Heimlich maneuver, and when is it used?

- It's used to clear a blocked airway in a choking victim by applying abdominal thrusts.

30. How should a CNA assist a patient with an IV infusion?

- Monitor the IV site for signs of infection, report any issues, and assist with dressing changes.

31. What is the purpose of oxygen therapy, and how is it administered?

- To improve oxygen levels in patients with respiratory issues; it can be administered via nasal cannula, mask, or ventilator.

32. How should a CNA assist a patient with a colostomy or ileostomy?

  - Provide care for the stoma, change the appliance, and assess for any issues.

33. How should a CNA handle a patient experiencing a panic attack?

  - Stay calm, provide reassurance, and help the patient focus on their breathing.

34. What is the purpose of post-mortem care?

  - To prepare the body for viewing by family members, ensure dignity, and report the death.

35. How should a CNA respond to a patient's complaint of chest pain?

  - Immediately notify the nurse or healthcare provider and assist with necessary interventions.

36. What is the purpose of wound care, and how should it be performed?

  - To promote healing and prevent infection; it includes cleaning, dressing changes, and monitoring.

37. How can CNAs assist patients with diabetes?

  - Monitor blood sugar levels, assist with insulin administration, and educate on dietary choices.

38. How should a CNA assist a patient with a broken bone?

  - Immobilize the affected area, provide pain relief, and report the injury to the nurse.

39. What is the purpose of a urinary catheter, and how is it maintained?

- To drain urine when a patient cannot do so independently; it should be kept clean and sterile.

40. How should a CNA handle a patient experiencing a seizure?

- Protect the patient from harm, move objects out of the way, and stay with them until the seizure ends.

41. How can CNAs assist patients with mental health issues?

- Provide emotional support, engage in therapeutic communication, and report any concerning behaviors.

42. What is the Heimlich maneuver, and when is it used?

- It's used to clear a blocked airway in a choking victim by applying abdominal thrusts.

43. How should a CNA assist a patient with an IV infusion?

- Monitor the IV site for signs of infection, report any issues, and assist with dressing changes.

44. What is the purpose of oxygen therapy, and how is it administered?

- To improve oxygen levels in patients with respiratory issues; it can be administered via nasal cannula, mask, or ventilator.

45. How should a CNA assist a patient with a colostomy or ileostomy?

- Provide care for the stoma, change the appliance, and assess for any issues.

46. How should a CNA handle a patient experiencing a panic attack?

- Stay calm, provide reassurance, and help the patient focus on their breathing.

47. What is the purpose of post-mortem care?

    - To prepare the body for viewing by family members, ensure dignity, and report the death.

48. How should a CNA respond to a patient's complaint of chest pain?

    - Immediately notify the nurse or healthcare provider and assist with necessary interventions.

49. What is the purpose of wound care, and how should it be performed?

    - To promote healing and prevent infection; it includes cleaning, dressing changes, and monitoring.

50. How can CNAs assist patients with diabetes?

    - Monitor blood sugar levels, assist with insulin administration, and educate on dietary choices.

51. How should a CNA assist a patient with a broken bone?

    - Immobilize the affected area, provide pain relief, and report the injury to the nurse.

52. How can CNAs promote cultural competence in patient care?

    - Respect diverse customs, beliefs, and traditions, and ask patients about their preferences.

53. What are the signs of dehydration in a patient?

    - Dry mouth, dark urine, sunken eyes, and low urine output.

54. How should a CNA assist a patient with a nasogastric (NG) tube?

- Check placement, provide oral care, and monitor for any complications.

55. What is the purpose of an EKG (Electrocardiogram), and how is it performed?

    - To assess heart function by recording electrical activity; electrodes are placed on the patient's skin.

56. How should a CNA assist a patient with a tracheostomy tube?

    - Keep the tube clean and clear, monitor for respiratory distress, and assist with suctioning if needed.

57. What are the signs of a urinary tract infection (UTI)?

    - Painful urination, frequent urination, and cloudy or bloody urine.

58. How should a CNA assist a patient with a feeding tube (G-tube or J-tube)?

    - Administer formula, check for placement, and provide oral hygiene.

59. What is the purpose of a Foley catheter, and how is it maintained?

    - To drain urine from the bladder; it should be kept clean and sterile, and the drainage bag emptied regularly.

60. How should a CNA respond to a patient who is agitated or aggressive?

    - Ensure safety, stay calm, and report the behavior to the nurse.

61. What are the principles of body mechanics for safe patient lifting?

- Bend at the knees, keep the back straight, and use proper lifting equipment.

62. How should a CNA assist a patient with a wound vac (negative pressure wound therapy)?

   - Monitor the device, change the dressing as needed, and report any issues.

63. What is the purpose of a cardiac monitor, and how does it work?

   - To continuously monitor the patient's heart rhythm; electrodes are placed on the chest and connected to the monitor.

64. How should a CNA assist a patient with an ostomy (colostomy, ileostomy, or urostomy)?

   - Provide care for the stoma, change the pouch, and assess for complications.

65. What are the signs of a stroke, and how should a CNA respond?

   - FAST (Face drooping, Arm weakness, Speech difficulty, Time to call 911); call for immediate medical help.

66. How should a CNA assist a patient with a mechanical ventilator?

   - Monitor the machine, suction the airway, and report any alarms or issues.

67. What is the purpose of a PICC (Peripherally Inserted Central Catheter) line, and how is it maintained?

   - To provide long-term intravenous access; it should be kept clean and dressed properly.

68. How should a CNA assist a patient with a chest tube?

- Monitor the drainage, ensure a secure connection, and report any signs of infection or complications.

69. What are the signs of hypoglycemia (low blood sugar), and how should a CNA respond?

- Shakiness, sweating, confusion; provide a source of sugar and notify the nurse.

70. How should a CNA assist a patient with a wound that has staples or sutures?

- Keep the area clean, report any signs of infection, and follow the healthcare provider's instructions.

71. What is the purpose of a peritoneal dialysis catheter, and how is it maintained?

- To remove waste and excess fluids from the abdomen; it should be kept clean, and dialysis solutions should be administered as prescribed.

72. How should a CNA assist a patient with a Jackson-Pratt (JP) drain?

- Monitor drainage, empty the reservoir, and keep the drain site clean.

73. What are the signs of an allergic reaction to medication?

- Rash, itching, swelling, difficulty breathing; stop the medication and notify the nurse.

74. How should a CNA assist a patient with a ventilator-dependent respiratory condition?

- Monitor ventilator settings, provide oral hygiene, and suction the airway as needed.

75. What is the purpose of a central venous catheter, and how is it maintained?

- To provide access for medication administration; it should be kept clean, and dressings should be changed per protocol.

76. How should a CNA assist a patient with a wound that requires packing?

- Follow sterile technique, pack the wound as ordered, and document the procedure.

77. What is the purpose of a wound culture, and how is it collected?

- To identify the presence of infection; collect a sterile specimen using a swab or syringe.

78. How should a CNA assist a patient with a Jackson-Pratt (JP) drain?

- Monitor drainage, empty the reservoir, and keep the drain site clean.

79. What are the signs of an allergic reaction to medication?

- Rash, itching, swelling, difficulty breathing; stop the medication and notify the nurse.

80. How should a CNA assist a patient with a ventilator-dependent respiratory condition?

- Monitor ventilator settings, provide oral hygiene, and suction the airway as needed.

81. What is the purpose of a central venous catheter, and how is it maintained?

- To provide access for medication administration; it should be kept clean, and dressings should be changed per protocol.

82. How should a CNA assist a patient with a wound that requires packing?

- Follow sterile technique, pack the wound as ordered, and document the procedure.

83. What is the purpose of a wound culture, and how is it collected?

- To identify the presence of infection; collect a sterile specimen using a swab or syringe.

84. How should a CNA assist a patient with a chest tube?

- Monitor the drainage, ensure a secure connection, and report any signs of infection or complications.

85. What are the signs of hypoglycemia (low blood sugar), and how should a CNA respond?

- Shakiness, sweating, confusion; provide a source of sugar and notify the nurse.

Chapter 33

List of Questions and Answers (3)

What is the role of a Certified Nursing Assistant (CNA)?

- Answer: CNAs provide basic nursing care and assistance to patients under the supervision of licensed nurses.

2. What are some key qualities of a good CNA?

- Answer: Compassion, patience, excellent communication skills, and attention to detail.

3. How do you maintain patient confidentiality?

- Answer: By not sharing patient information with unauthorized individuals and only discussing it with healthcare team members who have a need to know.

4. What is the importance of handwashing in infection control?

- Answer: Handwashing helps prevent the spread of infections by removing germs and bacteria from the hands.

5. What are common signs of a patient experiencing pain?

- Answer: Grimacing, verbal complaints, restlessness, increased heart rate, and changes in vital signs.

6. Describe the proper technique for measuring a patient's temperature using a digital thermometer.

- Answer: Insert the thermometer in the appropriate location (oral, ear, or rectal), wait for the reading to stabilize, and document the result.

7. How can you ensure patient safety when transferring them from a bed to a wheelchair?

- Answer: Use proper body mechanics, ensure the wheelchair is secure, and check for any obstacles or hazards.

8. Explain the RACE acronym in the context of fire safety.

- Answer: RACE stands for Rescue, Alarm, Contain, and Extinguish/Evacuate. It is a protocol to follow during a fire emergency.

9. What is the purpose of documenting patient information in medical records?

- Answer: To provide a comprehensive and accurate record of patient care, which aids in communication among healthcare providers and ensures legal accountability.

10. How do you assist a patient with their activities of daily living (ADLs)?

- Answer: Help with tasks like bathing, dressing, grooming, toileting, and eating, while promoting independence and dignity.

11. What should you do if you suspect a patient is experiencing a medical emergency?

- Answer: Quickly assess the situation, call for help, and initiate appropriate first aid or CPR if necessary.

12. What is the proper technique for turning and repositioning an immobile patient in bed?

- Answer: Use good body mechanics, use a drawsheet if available, and turn the patient gently to prevent pressure ulcers.

13. Describe the steps for assisting a patient with ambulation using a walker.

   - Answer: Help the patient stand, position the walker in front of them, and assist with walking while maintaining stability.

14. What is the purpose of using a bedpan or urinal for patients who cannot get out of bed?

   - Answer: To provide a means for patients to eliminate waste while remaining in bed and maintaining comfort.

15. How can you assist a patient with dementia or Alzheimer's disease in a supportive and compassionate manner?

   - Answer: Maintain a calm and reassuring demeanor, use clear and simple communication, and engage in activities that promote mental stimulation.

16. Explain the concept of "patient-centered care."

   - Answer: Patient-centered care focuses on meeting the individual needs and preferences of the patient, involving them in decisions about their care, and treating them with dignity and respect.

17. What is the purpose of the Heimlich maneuver, and when should it be used?

   - Answer: The Heimlich maneuver is used to clear a blocked airway in a choking patient by applying abdominal thrusts. It should be used when a person is unable to cough or breathe due to an obstructed airway.

18. How do you prevent the development of pressure ulcers (bedsores) in bedridden patients?

- Answer: Regularly reposition the patient, use pressure-relieving devices, keep the skin clean and dry, and provide proper nutrition and hydration.

19. Describe the proper technique for providing oral care to a patient with dentures.

- Answer: Remove the dentures, clean them thoroughly, clean the patient's mouth, and reinsert the dentures.

20. What is the role of a CNA in assisting with medication administration?

- Answer: CNAs typically do not administer medications but may assist by reminding patients to take their medications and documenting their compliance.

21. How can you assist a patient in maintaining their independence while ensuring their safety?

- Answer: Encourage and support their efforts to perform tasks on their own while offering assistance as needed to prevent falls or injury.

22. What is the purpose of range of motion (ROM) exercises, and how are they performed?

- Answer: ROM exercises help maintain joint flexibility and prevent muscle contractures. They involve gently moving each joint through its full range of motion.

23. How can you communicate effectively with non-verbal patients, such as those with communication disorders or intubated patients?

- Answer: Use gestures, pictures, and written communication tools, and be patient and attentive to their non-verbal cues.

24. What is the role of a CNA during a patient's end-of-life care?

- Answer: Provide emotional support, ensure comfort, assist with pain management, and respect the patient's wishes and cultural beliefs.

25. How do you assist a patient with feeding when they have difficulty swallowing (dysphagia)?

- Answer: Follow the prescribed diet texture, ensure the patient is in an upright position, and give small, manageable bites with adequate time between them.

26. Explain the importance of maintaining a clean and organized patient environment.

- Answer: A clean and organized environment reduces the risk of infections, accidents, and promotes the overall well-being of patients.

27. What steps should you take if a patient falls?

- Answer: Assess the patient for injuries, call for assistance, and follow the facility's protocols for reporting and documenting the incident.

28. How can you assist patients in maintaining their privacy and dignity during personal care tasks?

- Answer: Close curtains or doors, provide a gown or cover, communicate respectfully, and involve the patient in decisions about their care.

29. Describe the proper way to transfer a patient from a wheelchair to a bed.

- Answer: Position the wheelchair close to the bed, lock the wheelchair brakes, assist the patient to stand, pivot and lower them onto the bed.

30. What is the purpose of a bed bath, and how is it performed?

- Answer: A bed bath is given to patients who cannot bathe themselves. It involves washing and drying the patient's body while they remain in bed.

31. How can you recognize signs of abuse or neglect in a patient?

- Answer: Look for unexplained injuries, changes in behavior, withdrawal, fear of specific individuals, or signs of neglect such as poor hygiene or malnutrition.

32. Explain the concept of "informed consent" and its importance in healthcare.

- Answer: Informed consent involves providing patients with all relevant information about a medical procedure or treatment so they can make an educated decision about their care.

33. What are some common signs of infection in a patient?

- Answer: Fever, increased heart rate, redness or swelling, pus or discharge, and changes in mental status.

34. How can you assist a patient with catheter care?

- Answer: Follow proper hygiene, clean around the catheter insertion site, and maintain a closed drainage system.

35. What is the role of a CNA in post-mortem care?

- Answer: Respectfully prepare the deceased patient's body, provide emotional support to the family, and follow facility protocols for documentation and disposition of the body.

36. Describe the steps for donning and doffing personal protective equipment (PPE) correctly.

    - Answer: Wash hands, put on gown, mask, goggles/face shield, gloves (in that order) for donning, and remove in the reverse order (gloves, goggles/face shield, gown, mask) for doffing. Proper hand hygiene should be performed after removing all PPE.

37. What is the purpose of a Foley catheter, and how is it inserted?

    - Answer: A Foley catheter is used to drain urine from the bladder. It is inserted through the urethra into the bladder and secured in place.

38. How do you provide oral care to an unconscious patient to prevent complications like pneumonia?

    - Answer: Perform frequent mouth care, keep the head elevated, and use a suction device to remove excess oral secretions.

39. How can you assist a patient with diabetes in managing their condition?

    - Answer: Encourage proper diet, monitor blood glucose levels, assist with insulin administration if needed, and report any unusual symptoms or changes.

40. What are some common signs of dehydration in a patient?

    - Answer: Dry mouth, dark urine, sunken eyes, lethargy, and decreased urine output.

41. Describe the steps for taking a patient's blood pressure using a sphygmomanometer and stethoscope.

- Answer: Inflate the cuff until the radial pulse disappears, slowly release the pressure while listening with the stethoscope, and note the systolic and diastolic readings.

42. How do you provide care for a patient with a wound or pressure ulcer?

- Answer: Follow the healthcare provider's orders for wound care, clean the wound, apply dressings, and monitor for signs of infection.

43. Explain the principles of body mechanics and their importance in preventing injuries.

- Answer: Body mechanics involve proper posture and movement to minimize strain and injury. They are essential for a CNA to protect both themselves and their patients.

44. How can you promote good nutrition for patients who have difficulty eating?

- Answer: Offer small, frequent meals, assist with feeding as needed, and encourage the patient to eat foods they enjoy within their dietary restrictions.

45. What is the purpose of a sterile dressing change, and how is it performed?

- Answer: Sterile dressing changes prevent infection and promote wound healing. They involve removing the old dressing, cleaning the wound, and applying a new sterile dressing.

46. How can you assist patients in preventing falls and accidents in healthcare facilities?

- Answer: Keep walkways clear, provide non-slip footwear, use bed and chair alarms when necessary, and assist with mobility as needed.

47. Explain the role of a CNA in preventing the spread of healthcare-associated infections (HAIs).

- Answer: Follow proper hand hygiene, maintain a clean environment, use appropriate PPE, and adhere to isolation precautions.

48. What is the purpose of a sitz bath, and how is it administered to a patient?

- Answer: A sitz bath is used to soothe and cleanse the perineal area. It involves having the patient sit in warm water in a specially designed basin.

49. How do you assist a patient with a colostomy or ileostomy?

- Answer: Follow the healthcare provider's instructions for care, change the ostomy bag, and provide emotional support to the patient.

50. What are the signs of impending labor in a pregnant patient, and how can you assist them during this time?

- Answer: Signs may include contractions, rupture of membranes, and bloody show. Assist the patient by providing emotional support and notifying the healthcare team.

51. What is the role of a CNA in post-operative care for surgical patients?

- Answer: Monitor vital signs, assess the surgical site for signs of infection or complications, and assist with pain management as directed.

52. How can you promote patient comfort when they are bedridden for extended periods?

- Answer: Provide frequent position changes, use pressure-relieving devices, keep the patient clean and dry, and offer emotional support.

53. Describe the proper technique for measuring and recording a patient's urinary output.

- Answer: Use a graduated measuring container to collect urine, record the amount, and note the color, odor, and any abnormalities.

54. How do you respond to a patient who is experiencing delirium or confusion?

- Answer: Reorient the patient to their surroundings, use clear and simple communication, and provide a calm and soothing environment.

55. What is the purpose of a TED hose (anti-embolism stockings), and how are they applied to a patient?

- Answer: TED hose help prevent blood clots by promoting circulation. They are applied by rolling them up the leg, starting at the ankle and moving upward.

56. Explain the principles of infection control and the chain of infection.

- Answer: The chain of infection consists of six links: infectious agent, reservoir, portal of exit, mode of transmission, portal of entry, and susceptible host. Infection control practices aim to break one or more links in this chain to prevent the spread of infections.

57. How can you assist patients with respiratory conditions, such as COPD or asthma?

- Answer: Encourage prescribed breathing exercises, assist with administering inhalers or nebulizers, and monitor for signs of respiratory distress.

58. What is the purpose of a 24-hour urine collection, and how is it done?

- Answer: A 24-hour urine collection helps assess kidney function. It involves collecting all urine output over a 24-hour period and storing it in a special container.

59. How can you promote skin integrity in bedridden patients?

- Answer: Perform regular skin assessments, keep the skin clean and dry, use pressure-relieving devices, and encourage proper nutrition and hydration.

60. Explain the concept of cultural competence and its importance in healthcare.

- Answer: Cultural competence involves understanding and respecting the cultural beliefs, values, and practices of diverse patient populations to provide effective and sensitive care.

61. How do you assist a patient with a tracheostomy tube?

- Answer: Maintain proper tube care, suction secretions as needed, and provide emotional support to the patient and their family.

62. What is the purpose of oxygen therapy, and how is it administered to a patient?

- Answer: Oxygen therapy is used to increase the oxygen levels in the blood. It can be administered through nasal cannula, face mask, or other specialized devices as prescribed by the healthcare provider.

63. How can you assist a patient with Alzheimer's disease in maintaining their daily routine and reducing anxiety?

- Answer: Create a consistent daily schedule, use memory aids, provide familiar and comforting items, and offer reassurance and emotional support.

Chapter 34

List of Questions and Answers (4)

1. What is the role of a Certified Nursing Assistant (CNA)?

   - CNAs provide basic patient care under the supervision of nurses.

2. What are some key qualities a CNA should possess?

   - Compassion, patience, communication skills, and attention to detail.

3. How can CNAs maintain patient privacy and dignity?

   - By closing curtains, using modesty blankets, and speaking discreetly.

4. What is the importance of handwashing in healthcare settings?

   - Handwashing prevents the spread of infections.

5. What is the proper way to wash your hands as a CNA?

   - Wet hands, apply soap, scrub for 20 seconds, rinse, and dry thoroughly.

6. What should you do if a patient falls?

   - Call for help, stay with the patient, and report the incident.

7. How should you communicate with a non-verbal patient?

   - Use gestures, facial expressions, and body language to understand their needs.

8. What is the purpose of a bedpan?

- To collect urine and feces from patients who cannot use a toilet.

9. How can you prevent pressure ulcers in bedridden patients?

- Repositioning them regularly and using pressure-relieving devices.

10. What is the Heimlich maneuver, and when should it be used?

- It's a technique to clear a blocked airway in a choking adult; use it when someone cannot cough or breathe.

11. How can you ensure patient safety when transferring them from a bed to a wheelchair?

- Use proper body mechanics and assistive devices like a gait belt.

12. What is the purpose of taking a patient's vital signs?

- To assess their overall health and detect any abnormalities.

13. What are the four vital signs?

- Temperature, pulse, respiration rate, and blood pressure.

14. What is a normal body temperature range for adults?

- 97.8°F to 99.1°F (36.5°C to 37.3°C) orally.

15. What is the normal heart rate (pulse) for adults at rest?

- 60 to 100 beats per minute.

16. How should you count a patient's respiratory rate?

- Count their breaths for 60 seconds while they are unaware.

17. What is blood pressure, and what do the two numbers represent?

- Blood pressure is the force of blood against the walls of arteries. The two numbers represent systolic (maximum) and diastolic (minimum) pressures.

18. What is the normal range for systolic blood pressure?

- Less than 120 mm Hg.

19. What is the normal range for diastolic blood pressure?

- Less than 80 mm Hg.

20. How should you assist a patient with activities of daily living (ADLs)?

- Help with bathing, dressing, grooming, eating, and toileting as needed.

21. What is the purpose of range-of-motion (ROM) exercises for patients?

- To maintain joint flexibility and prevent contractures.

22. How can you help a patient who is experiencing difficulty swallowing (dysphagia)?

- Follow a recommended diet consistency, assist with feeding, and ensure a safe eating environment.

23. What is the purpose of an indwelling urinary catheter?

- To drain urine from the bladder when a patient cannot do so independently.

24. How often should you provide oral care for a bedridden patient?

- At least every 2 hours.

25. What is the ABCDE assessment in nursing?

- Airway, Breathing, Circulation, Disability, and Exposure assessment to identify potential issues.

26. How should you handle a patient who is experiencing a seizure?

- Protect their head, move nearby objects, and place them on their side.

27. What is the purpose of restraints in healthcare, and when should they be used?

- Restraints are used as a last resort to ensure patient safety when all other alternatives have been exhausted.

28. What is the proper technique for measuring and recording a patient's urine output?

- Use a graduated container and measure the output in milliliters (mL).

29. How can you prevent infection transmission in a healthcare setting?

- By practicing proper hand hygiene, wearing personal protective equipment (PPE), and following isolation protocols.

30. What are the stages of grief, and how can you support a grieving patient?

- Denial, anger, bargaining, depression, and acceptance; offer empathy and a listening ear.

31. How can you assist patients with mobility issues to prevent falls?

- Provide ambulation aids, assess the environment for hazards, and offer support when needed.

32. What is the purpose of the Patient's Bill of Rights?

- To ensure that patients receive respectful and quality care.

33. What are advance directives, and why are they important?

- Legal documents that express a patient's healthcare wishes in case they become unable to communicate; they guide medical decisions.

34. How should you communicate with a confused or disoriented patient?

- Use simple language, maintain a calm demeanor, and provide reassurance.

35. What is the purpose of a care plan in nursing?

- To outline individualized care goals and interventions for each patient.

36. How can you promote good nutrition for patients?

- Encourage balanced diets, assist with feeding if necessary, and monitor food intake.

37. What are common signs of infection in patients?

- Fever, increased heart rate, pain, redness, swelling, and discharge.

38. What is the purpose of a urinary catheter care protocol?

- To prevent urinary tract infections and ensure proper catheter hygiene.

39. How should you assist a patient with a wound dressing change?

- Follow proper aseptic technique, clean the wound, and apply a new dressing.

40. What is the role of a CNA during a code blue emergency?

- Follow the designated code team's instructions, provide CPR if trained, and assist as needed.

41. How should you handle a patient's request for pain relief?

- Report the request to the nurse and follow their instructions for administering pain medication.

42. What are the common signs of dehydration in patients?

- Dry mouth, dark urine, sunken eyes, and low blood pressure.

43. How can you promote a safe and comfortable sleeping environment for patients?

- Ensure a quiet, dimly lit room, and address any discomfort or pain.

44. What is the purpose of a fall risk assessment?

- To identify patients at risk of falling and implement preventive measures.

45. How should you handle a patient who refuses care or treatment?

- Respect their decision, document the refusal, and inform the nurse.

46. What is the importance of documenting patient care accurately?

- It ensures continuity of care, legal protection, and quality improvement.

47. How can you assist a patient with respiratory difficulties?

   - Administer oxygen as prescribed, monitor breathing, and keep the airway clear.

48. What is the purpose of a medical history interview?

   - To gather information about a patient's medical background, allergies, and current medications.

49. How should you measure a patient's height and weight?

   - Use a calibrated scale and stadiometer, and record in pounds and inches or kilograms and centimeters.

50. What is the role of a CNA in post-mortem care?

   - Prepare the deceased, provide emotional support to the family, and follow facility protocols.

51. How can you assist a patient with dementia or Alzheimer's disease?

   - Use redirection techniques, maintain a consistent routine, and provide a safe environment.

52. What is the purpose of a Foley catheter?

   - To drain urine continuously and monitor urine output in critically ill patients.

53. How should you provide oral hygiene for an unconscious patient?

   - Use a swab or sponge to clean the mouth and keep it moist.

54. What is the purpose of the Omnibus Budget Reconciliation Act (OBRA) in long-term care?

- To establish standards for nursing home care and improve resident quality of life.

55. How can you help prevent the development of pressure ulcers in wheelchair-bound patients?

- Ensure proper cushioning and repositioning, provide skin care, and monitor for redness.

56. How should you assist a patient with a colostomy bag?

- Follow specific care instructions, empty the bag, and monitor for complications.

57. What is the purpose of infection control measures in healthcare?

- To prevent the spread of infections among patients and healthcare workers.

58. How can you maintain patient confidentiality and HIPAA compliance?

- Avoid discussing patient information in public areas and only share information with authorized individuals.

59. What is the role of a CNA in assisting with wound care?

- Follow the nurse's instructions, maintain cleanliness, and protect against infection.

60. How should you handle a patient who is exhibiting aggressive behavior?

- Stay calm, maintain a safe distance, and seek assistance from the nurse or security if needed.

61. What is the purpose of a bed alarm in patient care?

- To alert healthcare providers when a patient attempts to leave the bed unsafely.

62. How can you assist a patient with a hearing impairment?

- Use gestures, write messages, and ensure hearing aids are properly functioning.

63. What is the importance of proper body mechanics when assisting patients?

- It prevents injury to both the patient and the caregiver.

64. How should you document an incident or an accident involving a patient?

- Describe the event accurately, including the date, time, location, individuals involved, and any injuries.

65. What is the purpose of a sterile dressing change?

- To prevent infection and promote wound healing.

66. How can you provide emotional support to a terminally ill patient and their family?

- Listen empathetically, offer comfort, and provide resources for counseling.

67. What is the purpose of a bowel program for patients with spinal cord injuries?

- To regulate bowel movements and prevent constipation or incontinence.

68. How can you assist a patient with diabetes in managing their blood sugar levels?

- Monitor blood glucose as ordered, administer insulin or oral medications, and promote a balanced diet.

69. What are the signs of respiratory distress, and how should you respond?

    - Rapid breathing, cyanosis, and use of accessory muscles; provide oxygen and notify the nurse.

70. How should you assist a patient with a nasogastric (NG) tube?

    - Verify tube placement, administer prescribed medications or feedings, and monitor for complications.

71. What is the importance of cultural competence in healthcare?

    - It ensures that care is respectful and responsive to the cultural beliefs and practices of diverse patients.

72. How can you help a patient with a urinary catheter to prevent infection?

    - Maintain proper catheter care, keep the drainage bag below the level of the bladder, and maintain a closed system.

73. What is the purpose of the Minimum Data Set (MDS) in long-term care facilities?

    - To assess the needs of residents and develop care plans accordingly.

74. How should you assist a patient with a tracheostomy tube?

    - Monitor for signs of respiratory distress, suction as needed, and keep the stoma clean.

75. What is the role of a CNA in promoting a safe environment for patients?

- Identify and remove hazards, keep walkways clear, and assist with mobility as needed.

76. How can you assist a patient with Parkinson's disease in activities of daily living?

   - Provide assistance with mobility, eating, and dressing, and encourage regular exercise.

77. What is the importance of regular repositioning for bedridden patients?

   - To prevent pressure ulcers and improve circulation.

78. How should you assist a patient with a feeding tube?

   - Verify tube placement, administer prescribed feedings, and monitor for complications.

79. What is the purpose of a fall risk assessment in healthcare facilities?

   - To identify patients at risk of falling and implement preventive measures.

80. How can you provide emotional support to a patient who is grieving the loss of a loved one?

   - Offer a listening ear, provide comfort, and connect them with support resources.

81. What is the role of a CNA in emergency preparedness in healthcare settings?

   - Follow facility protocols, assist with evacuation if necessary, and ensure patient safety.

82. How should you assist a patient with cognitive impairment in activities of daily living?

- Use simple instructions, maintain a routine, and provide reassurance.

83. What is the purpose of a urinary catheter irrigation?

- To clear any blockages or obstructions in the catheter.

84. How can you assist a patient with a gastrostomy tube (G-tube)?

- Administer prescribed feedings, keep the site clean, and monitor for complications.

85. What is the importance of proper hand hygiene in infection control?

- It is the most effective way to prevent the spread of germs in healthcare settings.

86. How should you assist a patient with a PICC line (Peripherally Inserted Central Catheter)?

- Maintain the line's integrity, monitor for signs of infection, and follow specific care instructions.

87. What is the role of a CNA in maintaining patient records?

- Document care accurately, report changes in condition, and assist with charting.

88. How can you provide comfort to a patient who is experiencing pain?

- Administer pain medication as ordered, use positioning techniques, and offer emotional support.

89. What is the purpose of a gastrostomy tube (G-tube)?

- To provide nutrition and medication directly into the stomach.

90. How should you assist a patient with vision impairment?

- Describe actions and objects verbally, provide clear directions, and offer assistance as needed.

91. What is the importance of proper disposal of biohazardous waste in healthcare?

- To prevent the spread of infectious diseases and protect the environment.

92. How can you assist a patient with a hearing aid?

- Ensure the device is clean and functioning, assist with placement, and report any issues.

93. What is the purpose of a log roll technique when moving a patient?

- To maintain the alignment of the spine and prevent injury when turning a patient.

94. How should you handle a patient who is experiencing a panic attack?

- Stay calm, reassure the patient, and encourage slow, deep breaths.

Chapter 35

List of Questions and Answers (5)

1. What does CNA stand for?

    - Certified Nursing Assistant.

2. What is the primary role of a CNA?

    - To provide basic nursing care to patients under the supervision of registered nurses (RNs) or licensed practical nurses (LPNs).

3. What is the importance of infection control in healthcare?

    - Infection control is crucial to prevent the spread of diseases and maintain patient safety.

4. How often should a CNA wash their hands while providing care?

    - Before and after each patient interaction, and whenever hands become visibly soiled.

5. What is the purpose of taking a patient's vital signs?

    - To monitor their overall health and detect any changes in their condition.

6. What are the four main vital signs?

    - Temperature, pulse rate, respiratory rate, and blood pressure.

7. How should you measure a patient's temperature using an oral thermometer?

    - Place the thermometer under the tongue and instruct the patient to keep their mouth closed for accurate measurement.

8. What is the normal range for body temperature in adults?

- 97.8°F to 99.1°F (36.5°C to 37.3°C).

9. How should you measure a patient's pulse rate?

- Count the beats for one minute or 30 seconds and multiply by 2.

10. What is the normal range for an adult's resting heart rate?

- 60 to 100 beats per minute.

11. What is the medical term for difficult or labored breathing?

- Dyspnea.

12. How should you measure a patient's respiratory rate?

- Count the number of breaths in one minute.

13. What is the normal range for an adult's respiratory rate?

- 12 to 20 breaths per minute.

14. What is the role of the CNA in assisting with mobility and transfers?

- To help patients move safely and comfortably.

15. When assisting a patient with transferring from a bed to a wheelchair, what should you ensure is locked?

- The wheelchair's brakes.

16. What is a bedpan used for, and how should it be positioned under a patient?

- A bedpan is used for collecting urine and feces. Position it with the wider end at the patient's buttocks.

17. What is the purpose of catheter care, and how often should it be performed?

- To prevent infection and ensure cleanliness. It should be performed daily.

18. What should you do if a patient complains of pain during a procedure?

- Stop the procedure immediately, assess the patient, and report it to the nurse.

19. What is the purpose of turning and repositioning bedridden patients?

- To prevent pressure ulcers and promote comfort.

20. How often should you turn and reposition a patient who is immobile?

- Typically every two hours.

21. What is the proper way to clean and care for a patient's dentures?

- Remove and clean them daily with a denture brush and denture cleaner, and store them in a denture cup with water.

22. How should you assist a patient with eating if they have difficulty swallowing (dysphagia)?

- Offer small, manageable bites and encourage them to eat slowly.

23. What is the Heimlich maneuver used for?

- To clear a blocked airway in a conscious choking victim.

24. What should you do if a patient becomes unresponsive and is not breathing?

- Start CPR (Cardiopulmonary Resuscitation) immediately.

25. What is the purpose of bed rails, and when should they be used?

- Bed rails are used to prevent falls and should only be used with the patient's consent or when necessary for safety.

26. What is the correct way to document patient information?

- Use clear and concise language, record facts only, and follow the facility's documentation guidelines.

27. What is the chain of command in a healthcare setting?

- The hierarchy of authority and communication, usually starting with the CNA, then the charge nurse, RN, and doctor.

28. Why is it important to maintain patient confidentiality?

- To protect the patient's privacy and comply with healthcare regulations (HIPAA).

29. What should you do if a patient refuses care or treatment?

- Respect their decision, inform the nurse, and document the refusal.

30. What is the purpose of a bed bath, and how should it be performed?

- To clean the patient's body when they are unable to bathe themselves. Follow the facility's protocol, using warm water and soap.

31. What are the common signs of a urinary tract infection (UTI)?

- Frequent urination, pain or burning during urination, cloudy or foul-smelling urine, and fever.

32. How should you assist a patient with ambulation using a walker?

- Stand to their side, hold the walker firmly, and provide support as needed.

33. What is the role of a CNA during patient transfers using a mechanical lift?

- To assist with positioning and ensure the patient's safety.

34. What is the primary responsibility of a CNA in caring for patients with dementia?

- To provide compassionate care, maintain a safe environment, and promote their well-being.

35. How can you effectively communicate with a patient who has Alzheimer's disease?

- Use simple language, maintain eye contact, and be patient and understanding.

36. What is the purpose of compression stockings, and how do they work?

- To improve circulation and prevent blood clots by applying pressure to the legs.

37. How often should you check a patient's skin for pressure ulcers, and what are the early signs?

- Check every shift and look for redness, warmth, or changes in skin texture.

38. What is the purpose of a urinary catheter, and how is it inserted?

- It is used to drain urine from the bladder. It is inserted by a trained healthcare professional.

39. How should you provide perineal care to a female patient?

- Clean the perineal area from front to back with gentle, wiping motions.

40. What is the purpose of a patient care plan, and how often should it be updated?

- A care plan outlines a patient's specific needs and goals. It should be updated regularly or as the patient's condition changes.

41. What is the role of a CNA in recording and reporting a patient's intake and output (I&O)?

- To accurately measure and document the patient's fluid intake (oral, IV, etc.) and output (urine, vomit, etc.).

42. What is the purpose of range of motion (ROM) exercises, and when should they be performed?

- To maintain joint flexibility and prevent contractures. They should be performed as prescribed by the healthcare provider.

43. What is the proper way to transfer a patient from a wheelchair to a bed?

- Use proper body mechanics, ensure the bed is at a comfortable height, and use a transfer belt if needed.

44. What is the role of a CNA in post-mortem care?

- To provide respectful and compassionate care to the deceased, prepare the body for transfer, and assist with documentation.

45. How should you handle a patient's personal belongings and valuables?

- Respect their privacy and ensure their belongings are safely stored and labeled.

46. What is the purpose of a catheter bag and how often should it be emptied?

- To collect urine from a patient with an indwelling catheter. It should be emptied when it is one-third to one-half full.

47. What is the difference between a full bed bath and a partial bed bath?

- A full bed bath involves cleaning the entire body, while a partial bed bath focuses on specific areas.

48. How should you provide oral care to an unconscious patient?

- Use a soft toothbrush and mouthwash or moistened swabs to clean the mouth and teeth.

49. What is the CNA's role in promoting patient safety during a transfer or ambulation?

- Assess the patient's stability, use appropriate equipment, and provide assistance as needed.

50. What are the common signs of dehydration in patients?

- Dry mouth, dark urine, sunken eyes, and lethargy.

51. How can you help prevent the development of pressure ulcers?

- Regularly reposition immobile patients, keep their skin clean and dry, and provide appropriate support surfaces.

52. What is the purpose of oxygen therapy, and how should it be administered?

- Oxygen therapy is used to treat respiratory conditions. It should be administered as prescribed by a healthcare provider.

53. What should you do if a patient falls?

    - Ensure their safety, call for assistance, and follow the facility's protocol for reporting and documenting the fall.

54. What are the principles of body mechanics, and why are they important for CNAs?

    - Body mechanics involve using proper posture and techniques to prevent injuries while assisting patients with mobility.

55. How can you communicate effectively with non-English speaking patients?

    - Use a professional interpreter or communication tools provided by the facility.

56. What is the purpose of documenting a patient's pain level, and how is it measured?

    - To assess and manage the patient's pain effectively. Pain can be measured using a pain scale (e.g., 0-10).

57. What is the role of a CNA in assisting with wound care?

    - To help clean and dress wounds as directed by the nurse or healthcare provider.

58. What should you do if a patient refuses to take medication?

    - Inform the nurse, document the refusal, and ensure the patient understands the consequences of refusing medication.

59. How should you assist a patient with donning and doffing personal protective equipment (PPE)?

- Follow the facility's guidelines for proper PPE usage, including gloves, gowns, masks, and eye protection.

60. What is the purpose of a code of ethics for CNAs, and how should it guide your behavior?

- A code of ethics provides ethical guidelines for professional conduct and ensures patient welfare and dignity are upheld.

61. How can you prevent the spread of healthcare-associated infections (HAIs)?

- Practice proper hand hygiene, use PPE as needed, and follow infection control protocols.

62. What is the role of a CNA in assisting with catheter care?

- To maintain a clean and sterile catheter, ensure proper positioning, and monitor for complications.

63. How can you effectively communicate with a patient who has a hearing impairment?

- Use written communication, gestures, and ensure the patient has access to hearing aids or assistive devices.

64. What is the purpose of a fall risk assessment, and how is it conducted?

- To identify patients at risk of falling. It is conducted upon admission and routinely thereafter.

65. What are the common signs of a urinary tract infection (UTI) in elderly patients?

- Confusion, agitation, incontinence, and a strong urge to urinate.

66. How should you assist a patient with eating who has difficulty holding utensils?

- Offer adaptive devices, cut food into small pieces, and provide assistance as needed.

67. What is the role of a CNA in administering tube feedings?

- To assist with the feeding process, monitor for complications, and report any issues to the nurse.

68. What is the purpose of a bladder scanner, and how is it used?

- A bladder scanner measures the volume of urine in the bladder non-invasively.

69. How should you assist a patient who has just had surgery and is experiencing pain?

- Provide pain relief as prescribed by the healthcare provider and offer emotional support.

70. What is the purpose of post-operative deep breathing exercises, and when should they be performed?

- To prevent complications such as pneumonia. They should be performed frequently after surgery.

71. How can you ensure patient privacy and dignity during care?

- Close curtains, use blankets or gowns for coverage, and communicate discreetly.

72. What is the role of a CNA during a patient's admission to a healthcare facility?

- To gather essential information, orient the patient to their room, and assist with initial assessments.

73. How should you provide foot care to diabetic patients?

- Carefully inspect the feet for any signs of injury, clean them gently, and moisturize dry skin.

74. What are the common signs of a stroke, and how should you respond?

- Sudden weakness or numbness, slurred speech, and difficulty with balance. Call for emergency assistance.

75. How should you assist a patient with dementia who becomes agitated or aggressive?

- Use non-confrontational techniques, redirect their attention, and ensure their safety.

76. What is the purpose of a sitz bath, and when is it commonly used?

- A sitz bath is used to soothe and clean the perineal area, often after childbirth or for hemorrhoid relief.

77. How should you assist a patient who requires oxygen therapy while eating?

- Ensure the oxygen flow rate is maintained, and use caution to prevent fire hazards.

78. What is the purpose of post-mortem care, and how should it be performed?

- To provide respectful care to the deceased and prepare the body for transfer to the morgue or funeral home.

79. How can you ensure that a patient with a language barrier understands their care instructions?

- Use visual aids, demonstrate procedures, and involve a professional interpreter when necessary.

80. What should you do if you suspect a patient is being abused or neglected?

- Report your suspicions to the appropriate authority or supervisor as mandated by your facility's policies.

81. How should you assist a patient with an indwelling urinary catheter in maintaining hygiene?

- Clean the catheter tubing and the area around the catheter insertion site as per facility protocol.

82. What is the purpose of logrolling a patient, and when should it be done?

- To maintain spinal alignment and prevent injury when turning or repositioning the patient.

83. What is the CNA's role in preventing medication errors?

- Double-check medication labels, verify the patient's identity, and report discrepancies to the nurse.

84. How should you assist a patient with dementia who has difficulty recognizing familiar people or places?

- Use reminiscence therapy, provide comforting cues, and maintain a consistent routine.

85. What are the steps for performing proper hand hygiene?

- Wet hands, apply soap, scrub for at least 20 seconds, rinse thoroughly, and dry with a clean towel.

Chapter 36

List of Questions and Answers (6)

1. Q: What is the primary role of a Certified Nursing Assistant (CNA)? A: CNAs provide basic patient care and assist with activities of daily living.

2. Q: How should you greet a patient when entering their room? A: Greet the patient with a warm smile and introduce yourself by name.

3. Q: What are vital signs, and why are they important for CNAs to monitor? A: Vital signs include temperature, pulse, respirations, and blood pressure. Monitoring them helps assess a patient's overall health.

4. Q: How should you respond if a patient complains of pain? A: Report the pain to the nurse and document it accurately.

5. Q: What is the proper handwashing technique for healthcare workers? A: Wash your hands with soap and warm water for at least 20 seconds, scrubbing all surfaces thoroughly.

6. Q: What is the purpose of a bedpan and when should it be used? A: A bedpan is used for patients who cannot get out of bed to use the toilet. It allows them to eliminate waste while lying down.

7. Q: What is the role of CNAs during mealtime? A: CNAs assist patients with eating, ensure they have the correct diet, and report any difficulties with swallowing or food allergies.

8. Q: How can CNAs help promote patient mobility and prevent pressure ulcers? A: CNAs can assist with repositioning and encourage patients to change positions regularly.

9. Q: What is the importance of maintaining patient confidentiality? A: Patient confidentiality is crucial to protect their privacy and maintain trust in the healthcare system.

10. Q: How should CNAs respond to a patient who is anxious or upset? A: Provide emotional support, listen actively, and inform the nurse of the patient's emotional state.

11. Q: What is the Heimlich maneuver, and when should it be used? A: The Heimlich maneuver is used to clear a blocked airway in a choking victim. It should be administered when a person is unable to cough or breathe.

12. Q: What is the proper technique for transferring a patient from a bed to a wheelchair? A: Use proper body mechanics and assistive devices like a transfer belt to ensure a safe transfer.

13. Q: How can CNAs help prevent the spread of infections in healthcare settings? A: CNAs can practice proper hand hygiene, wear personal protective equipment when necessary, and follow infection control protocols.

14. Q: What is the purpose of a Foley catheter, and how should it be cared for? A: A Foley catheter is used to drain urine from the bladder. CNAs should ensure proper placement, keep the tubing clean, and empty the drainage bag as needed.

15. Q: What is the role of CNAs in monitoring and reporting changes in a patient's condition? A: CNAs should regularly assess patients, report any changes to the nurse, and document their findings.

16. Q: How can CNAs assist patients with impaired mobility in using a commode? A: CNAs can position the commode bedside, help the patient transfer, and provide privacy and support.

17. Q: What is the purpose of a bed bath, and when might it be necessary? A: A bed bath is given to patients who are unable to bathe themselves. It helps maintain hygiene and skin integrity.

18. Q: How should CNAs handle medications for patients? A: CNAs are not typically allowed to administer medications. They should report any medication needs to the nurse.

19. Q: What should CNAs do in the event of a fire or other emergency? A: Follow the facility's emergency procedures, assist patients to safety, and report the situation to the nurse or designated personnel.

20. Q: Why is proper documentation essential for CNAs? A: Documentation provides a record of care, helps track patient progress, and ensures continuity of care among healthcare providers.

Chapter 37

List of Questions and Answers (7)

1. Q: What is the primary role of a CNA? A: The primary role of a CNA is to provide basic care and assistance to patients or residents in healthcare settings.

2. Q: How should you greet a patient when entering their room? A: Greet the patient with a warm and friendly smile, introduce yourself, and address them by their preferred name.

3. Q: What is the importance of hand hygiene in healthcare settings? A: Hand hygiene is crucial to prevent the spread of infections and maintain patient safety.

4. Q: How can you assist a patient with activities of daily living (ADLs)? A: You can assist with ADLs by helping with tasks such as bathing, dressing, grooming, toileting, and feeding as needed.

5. Q: What should you do if a patient falls? A: Assess the patient for injuries, call for help, and follow facility protocols for reporting and documenting the incident.

6. Q: What are pressure ulcers, and how can you prevent them? A: Pressure ulcers are skin injuries caused by prolonged pressure on the skin. To prevent them, reposition immobile patients regularly and provide proper skincare.

7. Q: What is the purpose of taking a patient's vital signs? A: Vital signs help monitor a patient's overall health and include measurements such as temperature, blood pressure, pulse rate, and respiratory rate.

8. Q: How can you ensure patient confidentiality? A: Always protect patient information, avoid discussing it in public areas, and follow HIPAA regulations.

9. Q: What is the Heimlich maneuver, and when should it be used? A: The Heimlich maneuver is a technique used to clear a blocked airway in a conscious choking victim.

10. Q: How should you handle a patient's emotional distress or anxiety? A: Provide emotional support, listen actively, and inform the nursing staff or supervisor if necessary.

11. Q: What is the purpose of documenting patient care? A: Documentation is essential for maintaining a patient's medical history, tracking changes in their condition, and providing legal protection.

12. Q: What is the proper technique for transferring a patient from a bed to a wheelchair? A: Use proper body mechanics, assistive devices, and follow facility guidelines to ensure a safe transfer.

13. Q: How can you promote infection control in a healthcare setting? A: Follow standard precautions, use personal protective equipment (PPE), and practice proper hand hygiene.

14. Q: What are some common signs of dehydration in patients? A: Common signs of dehydration include dry mouth, dark urine, sunken eyes, and decreased skin elasticity.

15. Q: What should you do if a patient refuses care or treatment? A: Respect the patient's autonomy, document the refusal, and inform the nursing staff or supervisor.

16. Q: What is the purpose of range of motion (ROM) exercises for patients? A: ROM exercises help maintain joint flexibility and prevent muscle atrophy in immobile patients.

17. Q: How can you assist a patient with mobility and walking? A: Provide support as needed, use assistive devices like walkers or canes, and ensure a safe environment.

18. Q: What is the role of a CNA during a patient's end-of-life care? A: Provide comfort, emotional support, and maintain the patient's dignity and privacy.

19. Q: What is the difference between sterile and non-sterile techniques? A: Sterile techniques are used to prevent contamination in procedures involving body cavities or open wounds, while non-sterile techniques are used for routine care.

20. Q: How can you effectively communicate with patients who have cognitive impairments? A: Use simple language, visual aids, and maintain a calm and patient demeanor when communicating with patients who have cognitive impairments.

Chapter 38

List of Questions and Answers (8)

1. What is the role of a Certified Nursing Assistant (CNA)? Answer: CNAs provide basic patient care under the supervision of registered nurses or licensed practical nurses.

2. What are some common tasks CNAs perform? Answer: Tasks include bathing patients, assisting with mobility, taking vital signs, and providing emotional support.

3. Explain the importance of patient confidentiality. Answer: Patient confidentiality is crucial to maintain trust and protect patient privacy.

4. How should you handle a patient who refuses care? Answer: Respect their decision, inform the nurse, and document the refusal.

5. What are vital signs, and why are they important? Answer: Vital signs include temperature, pulse, respiration rate, and blood pressure; they help assess a patient's overall health.

6. Describe the proper way to take a patient's temperature. Answer: Use a thermometer orally, rectally, or axillary, following hygiene and safety protocols.

7. What is the normal range for adult body temperature? Answer: The normal range for oral temperature is around 97.8°F to 99.1°F (36.5°C to 37.3°C).

8. What is the purpose of hand hygiene in healthcare settings? Answer: Hand hygiene prevents the spread of infections and keeps patients and staff safe.

9. How often should you perform hand hygiene? Answer: Before and after patient contact, after removing gloves, and when hands are visibly soiled.

10. Define the term "bedridden." Answer: A patient who is unable to get out of bed due to illness, injury, or mobility issues.

11. What are pressure ulcers, and how can they be prevented? Answer: Pressure ulcers are skin injuries caused by prolonged pressure. Prevention includes repositioning, good nutrition, and skin care.

12. Explain the RACE acronym in fire safety. Answer: RACE stands for Rescue, Alarm, Contain, and Extinguish. It's a protocol for responding to fires in healthcare settings.

13. When should you use the Heimlich maneuver? Answer: Use the Heimlich maneuver when a person is choking and unable to breathe.

14. What is the purpose of a bedpan and how should it be used? Answer: A bedpan is used for patients who cannot get out of bed to use the toilet. It should be positioned correctly and cleaned after use.

15. Define the term "incontinence." Answer: Incontinence is the inability to control bowel or bladder function.

16. How can you maintain proper body mechanics while lifting a patient? Answer: Bend your knees, keep your back straight, and use your leg muscles to lift.

17. What is the purpose of a catheter, and how should it be cared for? Answer: Catheters are used to drain urine from the bladder. Proper hygiene and monitoring are essential to prevent infection.

18. What is the role of a CNA during end-of-life care? Answer: Providing comfort, emotional support, and maintaining dignity for the patient.

Chapter 39

List of Questions and Answers (9)

1. What is the role of a Certified Nursing Assistant (CNA)? Answer: CNAs provide basic patient care under the supervision of registered nurses or licensed practical nurses.

2. What are some common tasks CNAs perform? Answer: Tasks include bathing patients, assisting with mobility, taking vital signs, and providing emotional support.

3. Explain the importance of patient confidentiality. Answer: Patient confidentiality is crucial to maintain trust and protect patient privacy.

4. How should you handle a patient who refuses care? Answer: Respect their decision, inform the nurse, and document the refusal.

5. What are vital signs, and why are they important? Answer: Vital signs include temperature, pulse, respiration rate, and blood pressure; they help assess a patient's overall health.

6. Describe the proper way to take a patient's temperature. Answer: Use a thermometer orally, rectally, or axillary, following hygiene and safety protocols.

7. What is the normal range for adult body temperature? Answer: The normal range for oral temperature is around 97.8°F to 99.1°F (36.5°C to 37.3°C).

8. What is the purpose of hand hygiene in healthcare settings? Answer: Hand hygiene prevents the spread of infections and keeps patients and staff safe.

9. How often should you perform hand hygiene? Answer: Before and after patient contact, after removing gloves, and when hands are visibly soiled.

10. Define the term "bedridden." Answer: A patient who is unable to get out of bed due to illness, injury, or mobility issues.

11. What are pressure ulcers, and how can they be prevented? Answer: Pressure ulcers are skin injuries caused by prolonged pressure. Prevention includes repositioning, good nutrition, and skin care.

12. Explain the RACE acronym in fire safety. Answer: RACE stands for Rescue, Alarm, Contain, and Extinguish. It's a protocol for responding to fires in healthcare settings.

13. When should you use the Heimlich maneuver? Answer: Use the Heimlich maneuver when a person is choking and unable to breathe.

14. What is the purpose of a bedpan and how should it be used? Answer: A bedpan is used for patients who cannot get out of bed to use the toilet. It should be positioned correctly and cleaned after use.

15. Define the term "incontinence." Answer: Incontinence is the inability to control bowel or bladder function.

16. How can you maintain proper body mechanics while lifting a patient? Answer: Bend your knees, keep your back straight, and use your leg muscles to lift.

17. What is the purpose of a catheter, and how should it be cared for? Answer: Catheters are used to drain urine from the bladder. Proper hygiene and monitoring are essential to prevent infection.

18. What is the role of a CNA during end-of-life care? Answer: Providing comfort, emotional support, and maintaining dignity for the patient.

Chapter 40

List of Questions and Answers (10)

Creating a list of 100 questions and answers for a Certified Nursing Assistant (CNA) book is quite extensive, but I can provide you with a sample of 20 questions and answers to get you started. You can expand on these and add more questions as needed:

1. Q: What is the role of a Certified Nursing Assistant (CNA)? A: CNAs provide direct care to patients or residents in healthcare settings, assisting with activities of daily living and ensuring their comfort and well-being.

2. Q: What is the difference between a CNA and an LPN (Licensed Practical Nurse)? A: CNAs assist with basic care tasks, while LPNs have more advanced training and can administer medication and perform additional nursing duties.

3. Q: How do you measure a patient's vital signs? A: Vital signs include temperature, pulse rate, respiration rate, and blood pressure. They are typically measured using appropriate instruments and techniques.

4. Q: What is the proper procedure for assisting a patient with bathing and personal hygiene? A: Maintain privacy, use warm water, provide a safe environment, and assist the patient as needed while respecting their dignity.

5. Q: How should you handle a patient with Alzheimer's disease or dementia? A: Approach them calmly, use clear and simple language, provide routine and consistency, and ensure their safety.

6. Q: What is the purpose of range of motion (ROM) exercises? A: ROM exercises help maintain joint flexibility, prevent contractures, and improve circulation for patients who have limited mobility.

7. Q: How do you properly transfer a patient from a bed to a wheelchair? A: Use proper body mechanics, use a transfer belt if available, and ensure the patient's safety throughout the process.

8. Q: What are the signs of a urinary tract infection (UTI) in a patient? A: Common signs include frequent urination, pain or burning during urination, cloudy or bloody urine, and fever.

9. Q: What is the purpose of turning and repositioning immobile patients? A: Regular turning and repositioning prevent pressure ulcers (bedsores) and promote comfort and circulation.

10. Q: How should you respond if a patient falls? A: Ensure their safety, call for help if needed, assess for injuries, and document the incident.

11. Q: What are the principles of infection control in a healthcare setting? A: Proper handwashing, using personal protective equipment (PPE), maintaining cleanliness, and following standard precautions.

12. Q: How do you assist a patient with eating who has difficulty swallowing (dysphagia)? A: Modify the diet consistency as recommended by the speech therapist, sit the patient upright, and provide small, manageable bites.

13. Q: What is the purpose of a bedpan or a urinal? A: Bedpans and urinals allow patients to eliminate waste when they cannot easily get out of bed.

14. Q: How do you handle a combative or agitated patient? A: Ensure safety for both the patient and yourself, use de-escalation techniques, and involve other staff as necessary.

15. Q: What is the role of a CNA in documenting patient information? A: CNAs should accurately document vital signs, care provided, changes in condition, and any significant observations in the patient's chart.

16. Q: What is the proper technique for providing mouth care to a patient?
    A: Use a soft toothbrush, clean the mouth, gums, and tongue, and ensure the patient rinses their mouth afterward.

17. Q: What is the difference between sterile and non-sterile techniques?
    A: Sterile techniques involve maintaining a completely germ-free environment, while non-sterile techniques focus on cleanliness but do not guarantee sterility.

18. Q: How do you assist a patient with a colostomy or ileostomy bag? A: Empty and clean the bag as needed, ensure proper placement, and provide emotional support to the patient.

19. Q: What should you do if you suspect a patient is experiencing a heart attack or stroke? A: Call 911 immediately, keep the patient calm and comfortable, and monitor their vital signs.

20. Q: How do you maintain patient confidentiality and privacy? A: Always keep patient information confidential, knock before entering a room, and only share patient information with authorized personnel.

Chapter 41

List of Questions and Answers (11)

1. What is the role of a Certified Nursing Assistant (CNA)? Answer: CNAs provide basic care and assistance to patients in healthcare settings, such as nursing homes and hospitals.

2. What are the key qualities of a good CNA? Answer: Compassion, patience, empathy, good communication skills, and attention to detail.

3. How can you maintain patient privacy and confidentiality? Answer: Always close curtains or doors, avoid discussing patient information in public areas, and follow facility policies.

4. What is the importance of hand hygiene in healthcare? Answer: Hand hygiene prevents the spread of infections and keeps patients safe.

5. How often should you wash your hands while working as a CNA? Answer: Before and after patient contact, after using the restroom, and before handling food.

6. What is the purpose of vital signs monitoring? Answer: To assess a patient's overall health and detect any changes that may require medical attention.

7. What are the four main vital signs? Answer: Temperature, pulse rate, respiratory rate, and blood pressure.

8. How do you measure a patient's temperature orally? Answer: Place a thermometer under the tongue and instruct the patient to keep their mouth closed for accurate measurement.

9. What is a normal adult body temperature range? Answer: 97.8°F to 99.1°F (36.5°C to 37.3°C).

10. How can you help a patient who is experiencing shortness of breath? Answer: Assist them to a comfortable position, encourage slow and deep breaths, and notify the nurse.

11. What should you do if a patient falls? Answer: Assess the patient for injuries, call for help, and report the incident to the nurse.

12. Describe the proper way to assist a patient with ambulation. Answer: Ensure the patient has proper footwear, use gait belts if necessary, and provide support as they walk.

13. How do you prevent pressure ulcers (bedsores)? Answer: Regularly reposition immobile patients, keep skin clean and dry, and provide good nutrition.

14. What is the Heimlich maneuver, and when is it used? Answer: It is a technique used to clear a blocked airway, typically when a person is choking.

15. How should you communicate with a patient who has dementia? Answer: Use simple and clear language, maintain eye contact, and be patient and understanding.

16. What is the purpose of range of motion (ROM) exercises? Answer: To maintain or improve a patient's joint flexibility and prevent muscle contractures.

17. How can you promote patient independence in daily activities? Answer: Encourage patients to do as much for themselves as possible, with your assistance when needed.

18. What is the role of a CNA during end-of-life care? Answer: Provide emotional support, keep the patient comfortable, and assist with their personal and spiritual needs.

19. How should you handle a patient's refusal of care? Answer: Respect their choice, document the refusal, and inform the nurse.

20. What is the purpose of the Omnibus Budget Reconciliation Act (OBRA)? Answer: It sets federal regulations for nursing homes and ensures quality care for residents.

21. What is the chain of command in healthcare? Answer: It is the hierarchy of authority, with the physician or nurse as the primary decision-makers.

22. How do you properly transfer a patient from a bed to a wheelchair? Answer: Use proper body mechanics, ensure the wheelchair is secure, and assist the patient in a safe manner.

23. What is the role of a CNA during emergency situations? Answer: Follow facility protocols, provide assistance to patients, and report the situation to the nurse.

24. What is the importance of documenting patient care? Answer: It provides a record of care provided, helps with communication among healthcare professionals, and ensures legal protection.

25. How often should you turn and reposition an immobilized patient to prevent pressure ulcers? Answer: Every 2 hours or as specified in the care plan.

26. What is the purpose of a catheter, and how should you care for a patient with one? Answer: Catheters are used to drain urine from the bladder. Care involves maintaining cleanliness and monitoring for infection.

27. What are the signs of infection in a wound? Answer: Redness, swelling, warmth, pain, and pus drainage.

28. How can you assist a patient with their daily oral care? Answer: Provide a toothbrush, toothpaste, and assist with brushing and rinsing as needed.

29. What is the purpose of a bedpan, and how should it be used? Answer: A bedpan is used for patients who cannot get out of bed to use the toilet. Position it correctly and provide privacy.

30. How do you help a patient who is experiencing incontinence? Answer: Change soiled linens promptly, provide clean clothing, and maintain dignity and privacy.

31. What is the proper technique for providing perineal care (peri-care)? Answer: Clean the perineal area from front to back using gentle, thorough strokes.

32. How can you ensure a safe environment for patients with dementia? Answer: Remove tripping hazards, secure wandering patients, and maintain a consistent daily routine.

33. What is the purpose of a Foley catheter, and how is it inserted? Answer: A Foley catheter is used for long-term urinary drainage. It is inserted through the urethra or a surgically created opening.

34. What is the purpose of oxygen therapy, and how do you administer it? Answer: Oxygen therapy provides supplemental oxygen to patients with respiratory issues. Follow the physician's orders and use the appropriate equipment.

35. How do you assist a patient with eating who has difficulty swallowing? Answer: Provide modified textures and small, manageable bites. Ensure they are sitting upright during meals.

36. What is the role of a CNA when a patient is receiving medication? Answer: Assist with medication reminders, ensure the patient takes the correct dose, and report any adverse reactions.

37. How should you handle a patient's emotional distress or anxiety? Answer: Provide a calm and supportive presence, listen actively, and report concerns to the nurse.

38. What is the purpose of restraints, and when can they be used? Answer: Restraints are used to prevent a patient from harming themselves or others. They should only be used as a last resort, with a physician's order, and in accordance with regulations.

39. How should you communicate with patients who have hearing impairments? Answer: Speak clearly and face the patient, use written communication if necessary, and provide hearing aids or other assistive devices.

40. What is the correct way to measure a patient's blood pressure? Answer: Use a properly calibrated sphygmomanometer, place the cuff on the patient's upper arm, and follow the correct technique for inflation and deflation.

41. What is the normal range for systolic and diastolic blood pressure in adults? Answer: Normal blood pressure is typically around 120/80 mm Hg.

42. How do you assist a patient with a walker or cane? Answer: Ensure the device is properly adjusted, provide stability and support as needed, and encourage proper posture.

43. What is the purpose of a sterile dressing change? Answer: To prevent infection and promote wound healing.

44. How should you provide oral care for an unconscious patient? Answer: Use a sponge swab or oral suction, be gentle, and ensure the patient's airway is clear.

45. How do you respond to a patient who is experiencing chest pain or discomfort? Answer: Notify the nurse or physician immediately, keep the patient calm, and assist with prescribed interventions.

46. What is the purpose of a tracheostomy tube, and how should it be cared for? Answer: A tracheostomy tube is used to maintain an open airway. Care involves cleaning the site and ensuring proper function.

47. How can you prevent falls in a healthcare setting? Answer: Keep the environment clutter-free, provide non-slip footwear, and use bed and chair alarms when necessary.

48. What is the role of a CNA in post-mortem care? Answer: Provide respectful care to the deceased, ensure proper documentation, and support grieving family members.

49. How should you handle and dispose of biohazardous waste? Answer: Follow facility protocols, use appropriate personal protective equipment (PPE), and dispose of waste in designated containers.

50. What is the purpose of a Foley catheter, and how is it removed? Answer: A Foley catheter is used for long-term urinary drainage. Removal involves deflating the balloon and gently withdrawing the catheter.

51. How should you assist a patient with a bedpan or urinal? Answer: Ensure privacy, position the bedpan or urinal correctly, and provide support as needed.

52. What is the importance of regular turning and repositioning for immobile patients? Answer: It helps prevent pressure ulcers and promotes comfort and circulation.

53. How can you promote oral hygiene for patients who are unable to brush their teeth? Answer: Use a moistened toothbrush or sponge swab to clean the mouth and teeth.

54. What is the purpose of a sitz bath, and how is it administered? Answer: A sitz bath is used to soothe perineal discomfort. It involves immersing the lower body in warm water for 15-20 minutes.

55. How do you assist a patient with a walker on stairs? Answer: Instruct the patient to use the handrails and lead with the strong leg when ascending and the weak leg when descending.

56. What is the purpose of a nasogastric (NG) tube, and how is it cared for? Answer: An NG tube is used for feeding or drainage. Care involves checking placement, monitoring for complications, and providing oral care.

57. How should you respond to a patient experiencing a seizure? Answer: Protect the patient from injury by moving objects away, place them on their side, and provide reassurance.

58. What is the importance of proper body mechanics for a CNA? Answer: It helps prevent injuries and strain while providing care to patients.

59. How should you assist a patient who needs to use a bedpan but cannot lift their hips? Answer: Use proper body mechanics and ask for assistance from another staff member if necessary.

60. What is the role of a CNA in infection control? Answer: Follow hand hygiene protocols, use personal protective equipment (PPE), and maintain a clean environment.

61. How can you help a patient with diabetes manage their condition? Answer: Assist with monitoring blood glucose levels, administer insulin as ordered, and encourage a balanced diet.

62. What is the purpose of a gastrostomy tube (G-tube), and how is it cared for? Answer: A G-tube provides direct access to the stomach for feeding. Care involves checking placement, administering feedings, and maintaining cleanliness.

63. How should you handle a patient who exhibits aggressive behavior? Answer: Ensure your safety and the safety of others, avoid confrontation, and notify the nurse or supervisor.

64. What is the purpose of a rectal tube, and how is it cared for? Answer: A rectal tube is used for the removal of flatus (gas). Care involves lubrication, insertion, and monitoring for complications.

65. How should you assist a patient with vision impairment? Answer: Use verbal cues, offer assistance with mobility, and ensure the environment is well-lit and free of obstacles.

66. What is the purpose of a stoma, and how should it be cared for? Answer: A stoma is an artificial opening created during surgery, often for colostomies or ileostomies. Care involves cleaning and protecting the area.

67. How can you help a patient who is experiencing constipation? Answer: Encourage a high-fiber diet, increase fluid intake, and monitor bowel movements.

68. What is the role of a CNA in wound care? Answer: Assist with dressing changes, observe for signs of infection, and report any concerns to the nurse.

69. How should you assist a patient with a wheelchair in a vehicle? Answer: Ensure proper positioning and secure the wheelchair using the vehicle's safety restraints.

70. What is the importance of documenting a patient's fluid intake and output? Answer: It helps assess hydration status and identifies any imbalances.

71. How should you assist a patient with dementia during mealtime? Answer: Provide familiar foods, set a routine, and offer assistance as needed.

72. What is the purpose of a continuous positive airway pressure (CPAP) machine? Answer: It is used to treat sleep apnea and maintain airway patency during sleep.

73. How should you assist a patient with a feeding tube (PEG tube)? Answer: Administer prescribed feedings, check tube placement, and monitor for complications.

74. What is the importance of proper disposal of sharps (needles and syringes)? Answer: It prevents needlestick injuries and the spread of infections.

75. How do you assist a patient who is non-compliant with their medication regimen? Answer: Educate the patient about the importance of medication, involve the healthcare team, and document the patient's refusal.

76. What is the role of a CNA in documenting patient care? Answer: Record vital signs, changes in condition, and care provided accurately and promptly.

77. How should you assist a patient with a hearing aid? Answer: Ensure the hearing aid is clean, functional, and properly fitted for the patient.

78. What is the purpose of a chest tube, and how is it cared for? Answer: A chest tube is used to remove air or fluid from the pleural space. Care involves monitoring drainage and keeping the system sealed.

79. How do you assist a patient with a tracheostomy tube during suctioning? Answer: Follow sterile technique, provide oxygen as needed, and monitor the patient's response.

80. What is the importance of maintaining a patient's dignity and respect? Answer: It preserves the patient's self-esteem and contributes to their overall well-being.

81. How should you assist a patient with a walker on uneven surfaces or stairs? Answer: Provide support and guidance, and ensure the patient feels stable.

Chapter 42

List of Questions and Answers (12)

1. What does CNA stand for? Answer: Certified Nursing Assistant

2. What is the primary role of a CNA? Answer: To provide basic care and assistance to patients under the supervision of a nurse.

3. Define HIPAA. Answer: HIPAA stands for the Health Insurance Portability and Accountability Act, which protects patients' privacy and the confidentiality of their medical information.

4. How often should a CNA take a patient's vital signs? Answer: Vital signs should be taken according to the facility's policy, often at least once per shift.

5. What are the four main vital signs? Answer: The four main vital signs are temperature, pulse, respiration rate, and blood pressure.

6. How should you measure a patient's temperature orally? Answer: Place the thermometer under the patient's tongue and wait for a few minutes until a stable reading is obtained.

7. When should you wash your hands as a CNA? Answer: Before and after providing care to a patient and after any potential exposure to bodily fluids.

8. What is the correct procedure for turning an immobile patient in bed? Answer: Use proper body mechanics and assistance to turn the patient while minimizing friction and shearing forces.

9. What is the purpose of range of motion (ROM) exercises? Answer: To maintain joint mobility, prevent contractures, and improve circulation for patients who have limited mobility.

10. Define the term "incontinence." Answer: Incontinence is the inability to control bowel or bladder function, leading to involuntary leakage.

11. What are the stages of pressure ulcers, and how are they categorized? Answer: Pressure ulcers are categorized into four stages: Stage I, Stage II, Stage III, and Stage IV, with each stage representing increasing tissue damage.

12. What is the Heimlich maneuver, and when is it used? Answer: The Heimlich maneuver is used to clear a blocked airway in a conscious adult or child who is choking.

13. What is the purpose of a bedpan and how should it be positioned? Answer: A bedpan is used for patients who cannot use a regular toilet. Position it correctly under the patient to collect waste.

14. How often should you encourage deep breathing exercises in bedridden patients? Answer: Encourage deep breathing exercises every 2 hours to prevent respiratory complications.

15. What should you do if you encounter a patient who has fallen on the floor? Answer: Assess the patient for injuries, call for help, and follow facility protocols for documenting and reporting the fall.

16. Explain the concept of "patient-centered care." Answer: Patient-centered care focuses on the individual needs and preferences of the patient, involving them in decisions about their care.

17. What is the role of a CNA during the admission and discharge process of a patient? Answer: CNAs assist with the admission process by gathering patient information and preparing the patient's room. During discharge, they help the patient gather belongings and provide instructions for follow-up care.

18. How should you position a patient with a nasogastric (NG) tube? Answer: The head of the bed should be elevated to prevent reflux, and

the patient's head should be turned to the side to minimize the risk of aspiration.

19. Explain the importance of documenting patient information accurately. Answer: Accurate documentation ensures that the patient's condition, care, and treatment are well-documented for legal and continuity of care purposes.

20. What is the purpose of sterile technique, and when should it be used? Answer: Sterile technique is used to prevent contamination during invasive procedures or when handling sterile equipment and supplies.

21. What is a Foley catheter, and why is it used? Answer: A Foley catheter is a flexible tube inserted into the bladder to drain urine when a patient cannot do so independently.

22. How often should a patient's position be changed to prevent pressure ulcers? Answer: A patient's position should be changed every 2 hours, and pressure-relieving devices should be used when appropriate.

23. What is the chain of infection, and how can it be broken? Answer: The chain of infection consists of six elements: infectious agent, reservoir, portal of exit, mode of transmission, portal of entry, and susceptible host. It can be broken by using infection control measures such as hand hygiene, personal protective equipment (PPE), and proper cleaning and disinfection.

24. Define the term "ambulation." Answer: Ambulation refers to the act of walking or assisting a patient in walking.

25. How should you assist a patient with a walker? Answer: Stand behind the patient, offering support and ensuring they maintain balance and proper posture.

26. Explain the role of a CNA in documenting food and fluid intake. Answer: CNAs are responsible for accurately recording the amount of

food and fluids consumed by the patient to monitor nutritional intake and hydration.

27. What is the purpose of a urinary catheter bag and how often should it be emptied? Answer: A urinary catheter bag collects urine for patients with indwelling catheters. It should be emptied when it is half-full or according to facility policy.

28. Describe the correct handwashing technique. Answer: Wet hands, apply soap, rub hands together for at least 20 seconds, including between fingers and under nails, rinse thoroughly, and dry with a clean towel.

29. What is the difference between subjective and objective information in patient documentation? Answer: Subjective information is based on the patient's feelings, thoughts, and opinions, while objective information is based on observable facts and measurable data.

30. How should you respond to a patient who is experiencing chest pain? Answer: Immediately notify a nurse or healthcare provider and follow facility protocols for assisting patients in distress.

31. What is the purpose of the Braden Scale? Answer: The Braden Scale is used to assess a patient's risk of developing pressure ulcers based on several factors, including sensory perception, moisture, activity, mobility, nutrition, and friction/shear.

32. How do you measure a patient's pulse? Answer: Use your fingers (usually the index and middle fingers) to palpate the pulse at a pulse point (e.g., radial or carotid) and count the beats for 60 seconds or 30 seconds and multiply by 2.

33. Explain the significance of a "Do Not Resuscitate" (DNR) order. Answer: A DNR order is a legal document that indicates a patient's wish to not receive cardiopulmonary resuscitation (CPR) in the event of cardiac arrest.

34. What is a pressure-relieving mattress, and when is it used? Answer: A pressure-relieving mattress or overlay is used to reduce the risk of pressure ulcers by distributing weight evenly and reducing pressure on vulnerable areas of the body.

35. How should you assist a patient with eating who has difficulty swallowing (dysphagia)? Answer: Follow the patient's dysphagia diet and feeding techniques recommended by the healthcare provider, which may include modifying food textures or using thickened liquids.

36. Explain the importance of infection control in healthcare settings. Answer: Infection control measures are crucial for preventing the spread of infections among patients and healthcare workers, ensuring a safe and healthy environment.

37. What is the purpose of a urinary catheter? Answer: A urinary catheter is used to drain urine from the bladder when a patient is unable to do so independently, such as after surgery or in cases of urinary retention.

38. Describe the correct procedure for transferring a patient from a bed to a wheelchair. Answer: Use proper body mechanics, ensure the wheelchair is locked and positioned appropriately, assist the patient to a sitting position on the edge of the bed, and pivot them into the wheelchair.

39. How should you handle a patient who is agitated or displaying aggressive behavior? Answer: Ensure the safety of the patient and others, use calm communication, and report the situation to the nurse or supervisor.

40. What is the purpose of a catheter care procedure? Answer: Catheter care involves cleaning and maintaining the cleanliness of the urinary catheter and surrounding area to prevent infection and complications.

41. What is a Code Blue in a healthcare setting? Answer: A Code Blue is an emergency code used to alert healthcare providers that a patient requires immediate resuscitation and urgent medical attention.

42. How can you promote good hygiene and oral care for bedridden patients? Answer: Regularly provide mouth care, brush the patient's teeth, and ensure they have access to mouthwash or oral moisturizers.

43. Explain the importance of proper body mechanics for CNAs. Answer: Proper body mechanics reduce the risk of injury for both the CNA and the patient while promoting efficient and safe care.

44. What is the role of a CNA during the transfer of a deceased patient? Answer: CNAs may assist with post-mortem care, which includes preparing the body, documenting the time of death, and providing emotional support to the family.

45. How do you assist a patient with using a bedpan? Answer: Place the bedpan correctly under the patient, ensure their comfort and privacy, and assist them as needed during the process.

46. What is the purpose of the Nurse Aide Registry (NAR)? Answer: The NAR is a database that maintains information on certified nursing assistants, ensuring they meet the necessary requirements and have a valid certification.

47. How should you respond to a patient who is experiencing a seizure? Answer: Ensure the patient's safety by moving objects away from them, gently guide them to the floor if necessary, and protect their head. Do not restrain the patient and document the seizure.

48. Explain the concept of "patient rights." Answer: Patient rights include the right to informed consent, privacy, confidentiality, and the right to receive appropriate care with respect and dignity.

49. What is the role of a CNA in maintaining a clean and sanitary environment in a healthcare facility? Answer: CNAs are responsible

for keeping patient rooms and common areas clean, including regular cleaning and disinfection of surfaces and equipment.

50. Describe the proper technique for measuring a patient's blood pressure. Answer: Use a sphygmomanometer and stethoscope, place the cuff snugly around the upper arm, inflate the cuff, listen for the Korotkoff sounds while slowly deflating the cuff, and record the systolic and diastolic pressures.

51. How do you perform passive range of motion (PROM) exercises for a patient? Answer: Gently move the patient's joints through their full range of motion without the patient exerting any effort. Perform PROM exercises to prevent contractures.

52. What is a Code Red in a healthcare facility? Answer: A Code Red typically refers to a fire emergency, and staff members must follow the facility's fire safety protocols.

53. Describe the purpose of a nursing care plan. Answer: A nursing care plan outlines the individualized care goals and interventions for a patient, providing a roadmap for their care and recovery.

54. How should you assist a patient with dementia during mealtime? Answer: Use familiar utensils and foods, provide verbal cues and encouragement, and maintain a calm and patient approach.

55. What are the common signs and symptoms of a urinary tract infection (UTI)? Answer: Common signs and symptoms of a UTI include pain or burning during urination, frequent urination, cloudy or bloody urine, and lower abdominal pain.

56. Explain the concept of "standard precautions." Answer: Standard precautions are infection control measures that should be applied to all patients, assuming that every patient may have an infectious disease. They include hand hygiene, wearing personal protective equipment (PPE), and safe handling of sharps and contaminated materials.

57. What is the primary purpose of a bed bath for a patient? Answer: A bed bath is used to maintain personal hygiene when a patient is unable to bathe independently, promoting comfort and cleanliness.

58. How can you assist a patient with impaired vision or blindness? Answer: Describe actions and surroundings, provide clear verbal instructions, and assist with mobility and activities of daily living as needed.

59. What is the purpose of a call light for a patient? Answer: A call light allows a patient to request assistance from healthcare staff when they need help or have an emergency.

60. How should you handle a patient's personal belongings? Answer: Respect the patient's privacy and property, keep belongings organized and accessible, and document any valuables.

61. Explain the significance of proper hand hygiene in infection control. Answer: Proper hand hygiene is the most effective way to prevent the spread of infections in healthcare settings, protecting both patients and healthcare workers.

62. What is the role of a CNA during a patient's bath or shower? Answer: CNAs assist patients with bathing, ensuring their safety, privacy, and comfort during the process.

63. Describe the procedure for measuring a patient's respiratory rate. Answer: Count the number of breaths a patient takes in one minute by observing their chest rise and fall, or listening to their breath sounds using a stethoscope.

64. What is the purpose of a sitz bath, and when is it used? Answer: A sitz bath is used to soothe and clean the perineal area, often after childbirth or for patients with certain medical conditions.

65. How should you respond to a patient who is anxious or agitated? Answer: Provide emotional support, maintain a calm and reassuring demeanor, and communicate clearly to address the patient's concerns.

66. Explain the importance of proper nutrition for patients in healthcare settings. Answer: Proper nutrition is essential for promoting healing, preventing malnutrition, and maintaining overall health in patients.

67. What is the purpose of a catheter bag with a drainage tube? Answer: The catheter bag collects urine and allows for easy monitoring of urinary output for patients with indwelling catheters.

68. How can you assist a patient with limited mobility during a bed bath? Answer: Use proper lifting and positioning techniques, provide support for weak or immobile limbs, and ensure the patient's safety during the bath.

69. Describe the appropriate technique for donning and doffing personal protective equipment (PPE). Answer: Follow the facility's guidelines for putting on and taking off PPE, ensuring proper hand hygiene and minimizing the risk of contamination.

Conclusion

In "**CNA for All**," we have embarked on a comprehensive journey through the multifaceted world of Certified Nursing Assistants (CNAs). This book has explored the essential skills, knowledge, and attributes that make CNAs invaluable contributors to the healthcare field. From the fundamental principles of patient care to the intricacies of ethical decision-making, CNAs play a vital role in ensuring the well-being and comfort of patients.

Throughout the 42 chapters of this book, we have witnessed how CNAs are not just caregivers but also advocates, communicators, and empathetic professionals who make a significant difference in the lives of those they serve. We have seen how CNAs prioritize patient safety, foster cultural competence, navigate ethical dilemmas, and embrace technology, all while providing care that is both patient-centered and dignified.

The journey of a CNA is one of continuous growth and development. CNAs must adapt to the evolving healthcare landscape, stay updated with best practices, and pursue opportunities for specialization and advancement. Their commitment to self-care, disaster preparedness, and interdisciplinary collaboration further demonstrates their dedication to their profession and patients.

In conclusion, "CNA for All" is a testament to the indispensable role that CNAs play in healthcare. Their dedication, compassion, and unwavering commitment to the well-being of their patients make them true healthcare heroes. As they continue to learn, advocate, and grow professionally, CNAs ensure that the principles of care, dignity, and compassion remain at the heart of healthcare, enriching the lives of countless individuals and families.

ABOUT THE AUTHOR (1)

Early Professional Experience (August 2007 - June 2008): After completing her degree, Rose embarked on her professional journey. From August 2007 to June 2008, she assumed the role of Secretary Manager at Maximum koneksyon in Port-au-Prince, Haiti. During this time, she played a pivotal role in supporting daily office operations. Her responsibilities included managing company correspondence, automating office processes, enhancing operational efficiency, overseeing inventory management, and ensuring that the office's supply needs were met promptly and efficiently. Rose's dedication and attention to detail were evident as she meticulously coordinated logistics to verify delivery dates, improving overall efficiency within the organization.

Customer Service and Professional Growth (November 2007 - June 2020): Rose's professional journey took a significant turn when she transitioned into the realm of customer service. From November 2007 to June 2008, she served as a Customer Service Agent at Uni-transfert central office in Port-au-Prince, Haiti. In this role, Rose managed a high volume of inbound and outbound customer calls, demonstrating her excellent communication skills. She addressed customer inquiries, suggested suitable alternatives when products were unavailable, and provided attentive responses to customer concerns. Her dedication to customer satisfaction was evident as she actively listened to customer questions, concerns, and needs.

Rose's pursuit of excellence led her to seek further education and training opportunities. In May 2020, she achieved a Certificate in Procurement and Logistics from Disasterready.org in collaboration with the USA United Nations. This certification underscored her proficiency in procurement and logistics management, which would prove invaluable in her future endeavors.

Dedication to Healthcare and Education (October 2008 - March 2018): In October 2008, Rose embarked on a fulfilling and impactful journey as the Director of the Vocational School Department at Heartline Ministries.org in Port-au-Prince, Haiti. Her tenure in this role lasted until March 2018 and was marked by her unwavering commitment to education and program management. Rose took on a leadership position where she meticulously

164

planned education programs, set ambitious goals, ensured compliance with legal and program requirements, and adeptly managed program budgets.

Her role extended to evaluating and supervising educators, assessing their performance, and providing essential support. Rose continuously sought opportunities for growth and collaboration, a testament to her proactive approach to education. She maintained up-to-date knowledge, consistently met and exceeded workflow demands, and effectively handled all delegated tasks.

Expanding Horizons and Professional Development (May 2020 - August 2022): In May 2020, Rose achieved yet another milestone by earning a Certificate in Hospitality and Tourism Management from Florida Atlantic University (FAU) in Boca Raton, FL. This certification highlighted her proficiency in managing and enhancing the guest experience in the dynamic hospitality and tourism industry.

Her commitment to excellence led her to embrace new challenges. In October 2021, Rose embraced the role of a Barista at Starbucks, located within the Florida Hotel and Conference Center in Orlando, FL. Throughout her tenure, which lasted until July 2022, Rose showcased her proficiency in preparing and serving high-quality coffee and tea drinks. Her exemplary customer service, efficient equipment handling, and comprehensive knowledge of the menu contributed significantly to the café's success. Rose's dedication to maintaining health and safety standards further exemplified her commitment to excellence in every role she undertook.

The Journey Continues (August 2022 - Present): In August 2022, Rose Andree Marjorie Tocel joined The Palms of St Lucie West – Independent, Assisted and Memory Care in Port St. Lucie, FL, as a Certified Nursing Assistant (CNA). Here, she continues to demonstrate exceptional caregiving skills by assisting residents with mobility needs, monitoring vital signs, and ensuring their well-being through assistance with Activities of Daily Living (ADLs).

February 20th, 2022: On February 20th, 2022, Rose took on the role of a Medical Assistant (MA) at Florida Community Health Center (FCHC), further diversifying her healthcare experience and responsibilities.

Personal Qualities and Values: Beyond her educational and professional accomplishments, Rose Andree Marjorie Tocel is highly regarded for her personal qualities. She embodies integrity, empathy, and strong leadership skills, setting an exemplary standard for those who have had the privilege of knowing her. Rose firmly believes in the power of education to transform lives and the importance of providing exceptional customer service. These values guide her actions and decisions both in her personal and professional life.

Future Endeavors and Inspiring Journey: As Rose Andree Marjorie Tocel looks to the future, her unwavering determination, commitment to excellence, and adaptability will undoubtedly continue to lead her to new heights in her career and personal life. Her journey is an inspiration, characterized by a dedication to serving others and making a positive impact on the world. Her diverse experiences and versatile skill set make her a valuable asset in any professional setting. Rose's lifelong commitment to learning and personal growth is a source of inspiration to all who have the privilege of knowing her. Her journey is a testament to the potential for success and impact that can be achieved through dedication, hard work, and a commitment to excellence. Rose Andree Marjorie Tocel is a professional of unparalleled dedication and integrity, leaving an indelible mark on every organization and community she serves.

Arsene Junior Joseph, the author of "There is Hope," "Let's Try Jesus," "The Power of Imagination," "I Was Born for Greatness", "Truck Dispatching Master" "Devenez un Truck Dispatcher", "Retour A l'Agriculture en Haiti", "Mastering ChatGPT", "Wake Up" and "Increase Your Faith" is a multifaceted visionary with a remarkable journey encompassing diverse fields and a profound commitment to personal growth and community development. Hailing from the vibrant state of Florida, Arsene's life story is an inspiring testament to the pursuit of knowledge, creativity, entrepreneurship, and philanthropy.

A Lifelong Love for Learning

Arsene's journey into the world of knowledge commenced early in life. His profound love for reading led him to immerse himself in books, nurturing a voracious appetite for learning. This passion for the written word eventually evolved into a talent for crafting literary works, establishing him as an accomplished book writer and songwriter.

A Voice of Motivation and Inspiration

Arsene's gift for inspiring others is a central facet of his identity. He has embraced the role of a motivational speaker, sharing potent insights and empowering messages that guide individuals toward realizing their fullest potential. His speaking engagements have taken him across national and international boundaries, allowing him to connect with diverse audiences and disseminate his message of hope and personal development.

A Multifaceted Career

Arsene's professional journey is a reflection of his versatility and unwavering determination. He is not only a celebrated author and songwriter but also a thriving business owner. His entrepreneurial spirit has led him to explore various ventures, including MLM marketing, where he has achieved success through diligence and innovation.

In addition to his entrepreneurial pursuits, Arsene is a dedicated English teacher, imparting language skills and knowledge to others. His linguistic prowess extends beyond English; he is fluent in Spanish and French, enabling effective global communication and skilled translation services.

The Heart of a Philanthropist

Arsene's deep-rooted Christian faith has instilled in him a profound sense of philanthropy. He is committed to giving back to the community and actively supports charitable causes that align with his values.

A Handyman with a Heart

Beyond his intellectual pursuits, Arsene is a practical individual with a knack for problem-solving and assisting others. He has earned a reputation as a skilled handyman, always ready to lend a helping hand.

A Champion of Community Development

Arsene is not only passionate about personal growth but also community development. His dedication to this cause is evident through his involvement in various initiatives and organizations. He holds certificates in an array of fields, including fundraising concepts, business expansion, management strategies, community organizing, grant writing, and public-private partnerships, among others. His commitment to responsible leadership, transparency, and good governance reflects his belief in creating positive change at both local and global levels.

A Creative Soul

Arsene's creativity knows no bounds. In 2009, he had the privilege of collaborating with a renowned artist to write "Stop Boasting," a musical composition that resonated with audiences worldwide.

A Member of YLAI

Arsene is a proud member of YLAI (Young Leaders of the Americas Initiative), a prestigious program that empowers young entrepreneurs and change-makers to foster economic development and strengthen ties between the Americas.

Arsene Junior Joseph's life journey serves as a powerful example of the potential within each of us to lead a purpose-driven life. His dedication to learning, creativity, entrepreneurship, and community development embodies the spirit of a true visionary, inspiring others to follow their paths of growth and positive impact.

Arsene's deep and abiding love for Jesus Christ is a powerful testament to the transformative power of faith. His journey of devotion and unwavering commitment to Christ serves as an inspiration to many, reminding us of the profound impact that a personal relationship with Jesus can have on one's life.

Arsene's love for Jesus is not merely a superficial sentiment but a profound and life-altering experience. It's a love that has shaped his character, guided his decisions, and infused every aspect of his life with purpose and meaning.

SUMMARY

"CNA for All" is a comprehensive guide for individuals interested in pursuing a career as Certified Nursing Assistants (CNAs) in the healthcare industry. This book provides valuable resources and knowledge for CNAs at all stages of their careers, including aspiring CNAs, current CNAs looking to enhance their skills, CNA students in training programs, healthcare educators, healthcare managers, allied healthcare professionals, and even patients and their families.

The book covers a wide range of topics, including the responsibilities of CNAs, patient care, ethical and legal considerations, understanding medical conditions and pathologies, effective communication and collaboration in healthcare, and quality improvement and patient safety. Throughout the book, real-life examples, insights, and practical guidance are provided to help CNAs excel in their roles and provide compassionate, high-quality care in diverse healthcare settings.

"CNA for All" is a valuable resource that equips CNAs with the knowledge and skills they need to deliver exceptional care, promote patient well-being, and contribute positively to the healthcare team. It emphasizes the importance of professionalism, empathy, and continuous learning in the field of nursing assistance. Whether you are aspiring to become a CNA or seeking to advance your career in healthcare, this book serves as an essential guide to succeed in the rewarding field of Certified Nursing Assistance.

POSITIVE QUOTES

1. "Caring is at the heart of being a Certified Nursing Assistant."

2. "Every patient is an opportunity to make a positive impact."

3. "Compassion is the key to providing exceptional care."

4. "In the world of healthcare, kindness is a universal language."

5. "A smile is the best medicine you can offer."

6. "Patient care is not just a job; it's a calling."

7. "Every day as a CNA is a chance to be a hero."

8. "Your dedication makes a difference in patients' lives."

9. "The bond between a CNA and their patient is priceless."

10. "Empathy is the bridge that connects you to your patients."

11. "The work you do as a CNA is a testament to your heart."

12. "With every act of care, you are changing lives."

13. "Kindness is a gift you can give to every patient."

14. "In the world of healthcare, positivity is contagious."

15. "Your passion for caregiving is your greatest strength."

16. "Dedication and compassion are the cornerstones of CNA practice."

17. "Your care is the light that guides patients through their darkest moments."

18. "The best way to find yourself is to lose yourself in the service of others." —Mahatma Gandhi

171

19. "CNA: Care, Nurture, Advocate."

20. "In the field of healthcare, every small gesture counts."

21. "A great CNA knows how to turn empathy into action."

22. "Your hands heal, your heart comforts."

23. "CNA: Bringing comfort, one patient at a time."

24. "The power of healing lies within your hands."

25. "Each day is a new opportunity to make a difference."

26. "Patience is a virtue, especially in the world of caregiving."

27. "Your compassion is the anchor in the storm of illness."

28. "In the heart of a CNA, kindness knows no bounds."

29. "Caring is the art of making patients feel valued."

30. "Your care is a beacon of hope for patients and their families."

31. "A great CNA treats every patient like family."

32. "Caring for patients is not a duty; it's a privilege."

33. "In the world of healthcare, optimism is a lifeline."

34. "Every moment spent in caregiving is a moment well spent."

35. "You are the guardian of your patients' well-being."

36. "Your dedication to excellence shines through in your care."

37. "A CNA's compassion is the heart of healthcare."

38. "Your role as a CNA is a testament to your strength.

40 POSITIVE QUOTES TO INSPIRE AND UPLIFT YOU

1. "Believe you can, and you're halfway there." —Theodore Roosevelt

2. "Every day is a new beginning."

3. "You are stronger than you think."

4. "Challenges are what make life interesting; overcoming them is what makes life meaningful." —Joshua J. Marine

5. "Happiness is not something ready-made. It comes from your own actions." —Dalai Lama

6. "You are the architect of your destiny."

7. "Success is not final, failure is not fatal: It is the courage to continue that counts." —Winston Churchill

8. "Every accomplishment starts with the decision to try."

9. "Your life is your message to the world; make it inspiring."

10. "The only way to do great work is to love what you do." —Steve Jobs

11. "The best is yet to come."

12. "In the middle of every difficulty lies opportunity." —Albert Einstein

13. "You are capable of amazing things."

14. "Keep your face always toward the sunshine—and shadows will fall behind you." —Walt Whitman

15. "The future belongs to those who believe in the beauty of their dreams." —Eleanor Roosevelt

16. "You are never too old to set another goal or to dream a new dream." —C.S. Lewis

17. "Life is 10% what happens to us and 90% how we react to it." —Charles R. Swindoll

18. "The only limit to our realization of tomorrow will be our doubts of today." —Franklin D. Roosevelt

19. "Every moment is a fresh beginning." —T.S. Eliot

20. "Dream big and dare to fail." —Norman Vaughan

21. "Today is your opportunity to build the tomorrow you want."

22. "The greatest glory in living lies not in never falling, but in rising every time we fall." —Nelson Mandela

23. "Don't count the days; make the days count." —Muhammad Ali

24. "Be yourself; everyone else is already taken." —Oscar Wilde

25. "You are what you believe yourself to be."

26. "The harder you work for something, the greater you'll feel when you achieve it."

27. "Happiness is an inside job."

28. "Believe in yourself, and you will be unstoppable."

29. "Do what you love, love what you do."

30. "Life is short, and it's up to you to make it sweet."

31. "Every day may not be good, but there's something good in every day."

32. "Your time is limited, don't waste it living someone else's life." —Steve Jobs

33. "Keep your head up, keep your heart strong."

34. "The journey of a thousand miles begins with a single step." —Lao Tzu

35. "The only person you should try to be better than is the person you were yesterday."

36. "Your attitude determines your direction."

37. "Don't watch the clock; do what it does—keep going." —Sam Levenson

38. "The secret to getting ahead is getting started." —Mark Twain

39. "Embrace the glorious mess that you are."

40. "You've got this."

May these quotes inspire and motivate you to live a positive and fulfilling life!

CNA GLOSSARY AND THE HEALTHCARE FIELD

1. **CNA (Certified Nursing Assistant)**: A healthcare professional who provides basic care to patients under the supervision of a licensed nurse.

2. **Patient Care Technician (PCT)**: Similar to a CNA, but with additional training that allows them to perform more complex tasks, such as EKGs and phlebotomy.

3. **ADLs (Activities of Daily Living)**: Basic self-care tasks, including bathing, dressing, eating, and toileting.

4. **HIPAA (Health Insurance Portability and Accountability Act)**: Legislation that protects patients' medical information and ensures its confidentiality.

5. **Infection Control**: Practices and procedures designed to prevent the spread of infections in healthcare settings.

6. **Nurse Aide Registry**: A state-run list of CNAs and other nursing assistants who meet state and federal training requirements.

7. **Scope of Practice**: The tasks and responsibilities that CNAs are legally allowed to perform, as defined by state regulations.

8. **Long-Term Care Facility**: A facility that provides care for individuals who are unable to care for themselves due to age, illness, or disability, over an extended period.

9. **Hospice Care**: Care provided to individuals with terminal illnesses, focusing on comfort and quality of life.

10. **Resident Rights**: The rights of individuals living in long-term care facilities, including the right to privacy, dignity, and autonomy.

11. **Vital Signs**: Measurements of basic body functions, including temperature, pulse rate, respiration rate, and blood pressure.

12. **Range of Motion (ROM) Exercises**: Exercises that help maintain or improve the flexibility of joints, often performed for patients who are bedridden or have limited mobility.

13. **Pressure Ulcer (Pressure Injury)**: A wound that results from prolonged pressure on the skin, often occurring in patients who are immobile or bedridden.

14. **Feeding Tube**: A tube inserted into the stomach to provide nutrition for patients who are unable to eat or swallow.

15. **Catheter**: A tube inserted into the body to drain urine from the bladder.

16. **Dementia**: A decline in cognitive function, including memory loss and reasoning, often associated with aging.

17. **Code Blue**: An emergency situation in which a patient requires immediate resuscitation, typically due to cardiac arrest or respiratory failure.

18. **Occupational Safety and Health Administration (OSHA)**: A federal agency that sets and enforces safety and health standards in the workplace, including healthcare settings.

19. **Personal Protective Equipment (PPE)**: Clothing and equipment worn to protect against exposure to infectious agents or other hazards.

20. **Advance Directives**: Legal documents that allow individuals to specify their wishes regarding medical treatment in the event they are unable to communicate them directly.

21. **Bloodborne Pathogens**: Infectious microorganisms present in blood that can cause disease, such as hepatitis B, hepatitis C, and HIV.

22. **Isolation Precautions**: Practices used to prevent the spread of infectious diseases, including wearing gloves, gowns, masks, and using special ventilation systems.

23. **Patient Transfer Techniques**: Methods used to safely move patients from one place to another, such as from a bed to a wheelchair.

24. **Resuscitation**: The process of reviving a person who has stopped breathing or whose heart has stopped beating, often referred to as CPR (Cardiopulmonary Resuscitation).

25. **Sterilization**: The process of killing all microorganisms, including bacteria, viruses, and fungi, on equipment and surfaces.

26. **Durable Power of Attorney for Healthcare**: A legal document that allows an individual to appoint someone else to make healthcare decisions on their behalf if they are unable to do so.

27. **Fall Risk Assessment**: An evaluation used to determine the likelihood of a patient falling and to implement measures to prevent falls.

28. **Gait Belt**: A device used to assist in transferring and walking with patients, providing support and stability.

29. **Hoyer Lift**: A mechanical device used to lift and transfer patients who are unable to move themselves.

30. **Tube Feeding**: The administration of nutrients directly into the stomach or intestines through a tube, bypassing the mouth.

31. **Disability**: A physical or mental impairment that substantially limits one or more major life activities.

32. **Palliative Care**: Care that focuses on providing relief from the symptoms and stress of a serious illness, with the goal of improving quality of life for both the patient and their family.

33. **Patient Advocacy**: The act of supporting and promoting the rights and interests of patients, ensuring they receive appropriate care and treatment.

34. **Restraints**: Devices or methods used to limit a patient's movement, typically used to prevent falls or to protect the patient from harming themselves or others.

35. **Resident Assessment**: An evaluation of a resident's physical, mental, and emotional status to develop a care plan tailored to their needs.

36. **Sepsis**: A life-threatening condition that occurs when the body's response to an infection causes inflammation throughout the body.

37. **Supine Position**: Lying flat on the back, facing upward.

38. **Prone Position**: Lying flat on the stomach, facing downward.

39. **Side-lying Position**: Lying on one side with the top knee bent and supported by a pillow, to prevent pressure ulcers and maintain comfort.

40. **Wound Care**: The process of cleaning, treating, and dressing wounds to promote healing and prevent infection.

41. **Ambulate**: To walk or move about.

42. **Assistive Devices**: Devices used to help patients with mobility or other activities, such as canes, walkers, and grab bars.

43. **Biohazard**: Biological substances that pose a threat to the health of living organisms, including humans.

44. **Charting**: The process of documenting patient information, including vital signs, treatments, and observations, in medical records.

45. **Cognition**: The mental processes involved in understanding and processing information, including memory, attention, and reasoning.

46. **Cultural Competence**: The ability to interact effectively with people of different cultures, understanding and respecting their beliefs, practices, and values.

47. **Dehydration**: A condition that occurs when the body loses more fluid than it takes in, leading to symptoms such as thirst, dry mouth, and dark urine.

48. **Hypertension**: High blood pressure, a common condition that can lead to serious health problems if left untreated.

49. **Hypotension**: Low blood pressure, which can cause symptoms such as dizziness, lightheadedness, and fainting.

50. **Medical Ethics**: The principles that govern the moral and ethical issues in healthcare, including patient confidentiality, informed consent, and end-of-life care.

51. **Necrosis**: Death of cells or tissues due to disease or injury.

52. **Orthostatic Hypotension**: A sudden drop in blood pressure that occurs when a person stands up from a sitting or lying position, causing dizziness or fainting.

53. **Pallor**: Unusual paleness of the skin, often a sign of illness or shock.

54. **Rehabilitation**: The process of restoring a person's abilities after an illness or injury, often through physical therapy, occupational therapy, or speech therapy.

55. **Respite Care**: Temporary care provided to relieve family members or other caregivers who are responsible for the ongoing care of a patient.

56. **Subacute Care**: Care provided to patients who are not acutely ill but require more intensive services than those provided in a skilled nursing facility.

57. **Tachycardia**: Abnormally rapid heart rate, often defined as a heart rate greater than 100 beats per minute.

58. **Thrombosis**: The formation of a blood clot inside a blood vessel, which can lead to serious complications if the clot breaks loose and travels to other parts of the body.

59. **Transcribe**: To write down or type out information from one form to another, such as transcribing a physician's orders or notes.

60. **Urinary Incontinence**: The involuntary leakage of urine, a common condition that can affect people of all ages.

61. **Afebrile**: Having no fever, or a normal body temperature.

62. **Auscultation**: Listening to sounds within the body, typically using a stethoscope, to assess the function of organs such as the heart, lungs, and intestines.

63. **Catheterization**: The insertion of a catheter into a body cavity or organ, such as the bladder, to drain urine or administer fluids.

64. **Decubitus Ulcer**: Another term for a pressure ulcer or bedsore, which is a localized injury to the skin and/or underlying tissue, usually over a bony prominence.

65. **Dysphagia**: Difficulty swallowing, which can occur due to various medical conditions or injuries.

66. **Emesis**: The act of vomiting or the material that is vomited.

67. **Exacerbation**: A worsening or flare-up of a disease or condition.

68. **Gastrostomy Tube**: A tube inserted through the abdomen into the stomach to provide nutrition or administer medications.

69. **Hemiplegia**: Paralysis of one side of the body, usually caused by a stroke or brain injury.

70. **Ileostomy**: A surgical procedure in which a portion of the ileum (the lower part of the small intestine) is brought through the abdominal wall

to create a stoma, allowing for the elimination of stool into a collection bag.

71. **Jaundice**: A yellowish discoloration of the skin and eyes caused by a buildup of bilirubin in the blood, often indicating liver or gallbladder disease.

72. **Lumbar Puncture**: A procedure in which a needle is inserted into the spinal canal to collect cerebrospinal fluid for diagnostic purposes or to administer medications.

73. **Malnutrition**: A condition resulting from inadequate intake of nutrients or the inability to absorb or use nutrients properly, leading to health problems.

74. **Nystagmus**: Involuntary, rapid eye movements that may be horizontal, vertical, or rotary, often indicating a neurological problem.

75. **Paracentesis**: A procedure in which a needle or catheter is inserted into the abdominal cavity to remove fluid for diagnostic or therapeutic purposes.

76. **Peristalsis**: The wave-like muscle contractions that propel food and waste through the digestive system.

77. **Phlebitis**: Inflammation of a vein, often accompanied by pain, redness, and swelling.

78. **Sputum**: Mucus that is coughed up from the lower airways, often used for diagnostic purposes in respiratory conditions.

79. **Thromboembolism**: The obstruction of a blood vessel by a blood clot that has broken loose from its site of formation.

80. **Vesicostomy**: A surgical procedure in which a small opening is created in the bladder to allow for the drainage of urine, often used in cases of urinary retention or dysfunction.

81. **Abduction**: Movement of a body part away from the midline of the body, such as moving the arm away from the torso.

82. **Adhesion**: Abnormal tissue attachment that can occur following surgery or injury, causing organs or tissues to stick together.

83. **Anaphylaxis**: A severe, life-threatening allergic reaction that can cause difficulty breathing, a sudden drop in blood pressure, and other serious symptoms.

84. **Anticoagulant**: A medication that prevents the formation of blood clots.

85. **Atelectasis**: Collapse or incomplete expansion of a lung or part of a lung, often due to blockage of the air passages or pressure on the lung.

86. **Dyspnea**: Difficulty breathing or shortness of breath.

87. **Electrolytes**: Minerals in the body that carry an electric charge and are essential for various bodily functions, including nerve and muscle function, and maintaining fluid balance.

88. **Embolism**: The sudden blockage of a blood vessel by a clot or other foreign material that has been carried in the bloodstream.

89. **Hematoma**: A localized collection of blood outside the blood vessels, usually caused by injury or surgery.

90. **Hypoxia**: A condition in which the body or a region of the body is deprived of adequate oxygen supply.

91. **Laceration**: A wound caused by tearing of the skin or other tissues, often with jagged edges.

92. **Myocardial Infarction**: Commonly known as a heart attack, it occurs when blood flow to a part of the heart is blocked, leading to damage or death of the heart muscle.

183

93. **Nasogastric Tube**: A tube inserted through the nose into the stomach to administer fluids, medications, or nutrition.

94. **Orthopnea**: Difficulty breathing while lying flat, often relieved by sitting or standing upright.

95. **Pneumothorax**: A condition in which air leaks into the space between the lung and the chest wall, causing the lung to collapse partially or completely.

96. **Purulent**: Containing pus, a thick, yellowish or greenish fluid that is produced in infected tissues.

97. **Sepsis**: A life-threatening condition that occurs when the body's response to an infection causes inflammation throughout the body.

98. **Stoma**: An opening created surgically on the surface of the body to allow for the drainage of waste, such as in a colostomy or ileostomy.

99. **Thrombophlebitis**: Inflammation of a vein that is associated with the formation of a blood clot.

100. **Turgor**: The elasticity or resilience of the skin, often used as an indicator of hydration status.

101. **Abdominal Aortic Aneurysm (AAA)**: A bulge or swelling in the aorta, the body's main artery, which passes through the abdomen.

102. **Abrasion**: A superficial wound in which the skin is scraped or rubbed off.

103. **Anemia**: A condition in which there is a lower than normal number of red blood cells or hemoglobin in the blood, leading to reduced oxygen flow to tissues.

104. **Aphasia**: A language disorder that affects a person's ability to communicate, often caused by brain damage from a stroke or injury.

105.   **Atrophy**: A decrease in the size or function of a body part, tissue, or organ, often due to lack of use or injury.

106.   **Bowel Obstruction**: A blockage in the intestines that prevents the normal passage of stool.

107.   **Cachexia**: A wasting syndrome characterized by weight loss, muscle atrophy, fatigue, weakness, and loss of appetite, often seen in patients with advanced cancer or other chronic illnesses.

108.   **Cathartic**: A substance that induces bowel movements and relieves constipation.

109.   **Decubitus**: Another term for a pressure ulcer or bedsore, which is a localized injury to the skin and/or underlying tissue, usually over a bony prominence.

110.   **Dysuria**: Painful or difficult urination, often caused by a urinary tract infection or other underlying condition.

111.   **Edema**: Swelling caused by excess fluid trapped in body tissues, often seen in the legs, ankles, and feet.

112.   **Erythema**: Redness of the skin, often caused by inflammation or infection.

113.   **Fecal Impaction**: A mass of hardened stool that cannot be passed from the rectum, often causing constipation and abdominal pain.

114.   **Hematocrit**: The percentage of red blood cells in the total volume of blood, often used as a measure of anemia or hydration status.

115.   **Hemoptysis**: The coughing up of blood or blood-stained mucus from the respiratory tract.

116.   **Irrigate**: To wash out a body cavity or wound with a stream of fluid, often to remove debris or infection.

117.	**Lumbar**: Relating to the lower back or the area near the waist.

118.	**Melena**: Black, tarry stools caused by the presence of partially digested blood in the digestive tract.

119.	**Occlusion**: The blockage or closure of a blood vessel or other tubular organ.

120.	**Paralysis**: Loss of muscle function in part of your body. It can be localized or generalized, partial or complete, and temporary or permanent.**Peritoneal Dialysis**: A type of dialysis that uses the lining of the abdomen (peritoneum) to filter waste and excess fluid from the blood.

121.	**Petechiae**: Tiny, pinpoint-sized purple or red spots on the skin caused by small amounts of bleeding under the skin.

122.	**Pruritus**: Itching of the skin, often caused by a skin condition or systemic disease.

123.	**Purulent Drainage**: Drainage from a wound or body orifice that is thick, opaque, and contains pus.

124.	**Renal Failure**: The loss of kidney function, which can be acute (sudden) or chronic (long-term).

125.	**Rigor Mortis**: The stiffening of muscles after death, which occurs due to chemical changes in the muscles.

126.	**Sclera**: The white outer layer of the eyeball.

127.	**Sepsis**: A serious condition that occurs when the body's response to an infection causes inflammation throughout the body.

128.	**Sinus Arrhythmia**: An irregular heartbeat that is normal in young people and can be influenced by breathing rate.

129.   **Sputum Culture**: A laboratory test used to detect and identify bacteria or other pathogens in sputum (mucus coughed up from the respiratory tract).

130.   **Stenosis**: The narrowing or constriction of a body passage or opening.

131.   **Stomatitis**: Inflammation of the mucous membranes of the mouth.

132.   **Suprapubic**: Located above the pubic bone.

133.   **Tinnitus**: Ringing or buzzing in the ears.

134.   **Tracheostomy**: A surgical procedure to create an opening in the neck into the trachea (windpipe) to allow for breathing.

135.   **Tympanic Membrane**: The eardrum, a thin membrane that separates the outer ear from the middle ear.

136.   **Urethra**: The tube that carries urine from the bladder to the outside of the body.

137.   **Vertigo**: A sensation of spinning or dizziness, often due to an inner ear problem.

138.   **Wheezing**: A high-pitched whistling sound that occurs during breathing, often due to narrowed airways.

139.   **Xerostomia**: Dryness of the mouth caused by reduced saliva production.

140.   **Anthropometry**: The measurement of the size and proportions of the human body.

141.   **Apgar Score**: A scoring system used to evaluate the physical condition of newborns at one and five minutes after birth.

142. **Asepsis**: The absence of bacteria, viruses, and other microorganisms.

143. **Ataxia**: Loss of full control of bodily movements.

144. **Catheter-associated Urinary Tract Infection (CAUTI)**: An infection that occurs in the urinary tract as a result of using a catheter.

145. **Cerebrovascular Accident (CVA)**: Another term for a stroke, which occurs when blood flow to the brain is interrupted, leading to brain damage.

146. **Deep Vein Thrombosis (DVT)**: A blood clot that forms in a deep vein, usually in the leg.

147. **Dysphasia**: Partial or complete impairment of the ability to communicate resulting from brain injury.

148. **Empathy**: The ability to understand and share the feelings of another.

149. **Endotracheal Tube**: A tube inserted through the mouth or nose into the trachea to maintain an open airway or to administer certain drugs.

150. **Epidural**: An injection of medication into the space around the spinal cord to provide pain relief.

151. **Erythematous**: Redness of the skin or mucous membranes due to dilation and congestion of superficial capillaries.

152. **Foley Catheter**: A type of indwelling urinary catheter that is held in place by a balloon filled with sterile water.

153. **Glasgow Coma Scale**: A neurological scale used to assess the level of consciousness in patients with brain injuries.

154. **Hypertonic**: Having a higher osmotic pressure than another solution.

155. **Integumentary System**: The organ system that protects the body from various kinds of damage.

156. **Lymphedema**: Swelling (usually in the legs or arms) caused by the retention of lymphatic fluid due to blockage or removal of lymph nodes.

157. **Narcotic**: A drug that relieves pain and induces sleep.

158. **Nystatin**: An antifungal medication used to treat fungal infections, such as oral thrush or yeast infections.

159. **Orthostatic Hypotension**: A sudden drop in blood pressure that occurs when a person stands up from a sitting or lying position.

160. **Palpitation**: A noticeably rapid, strong, or irregular heartbeat due to agitation, exertion, or illness.

161. **Paralysis**: Loss of muscle function in part of your body. It can be localized or generalized, partial or complete, and temporary or permanent.

162. **Paresthesia**: Abnormal sensations such as tingling, numbness, or prickling, typically due to nerve damage or dysfunction.

163. **Perfusion**: The passage of fluid through the circulatory system or lymphatic system to an organ or tissue, usually to provide oxygen and nutrients.

164. **Polyuria**: Excessive production of urine, often seen in conditions such as diabetes mellitus or diabetes insipidus.

165. **Pulmonary Edema**: A condition caused by excess fluid in the lungs, often due to heart failure or severe infection.

166.   **Pyrexia**: Another term for fever, an elevated body temperature often due to illness or infection.

167.   **Rales**: Abnormal crackling or rattling sounds heard when listening to the lungs with a stethoscope, often due to fluid in the lungs.

168.   **Renal Calculi**: Kidney stones, hard deposits of minerals and salts that form in the kidneys and can cause severe pain and other symptoms.

169.   **Seizure**: A sudden, uncontrolled electrical disturbance in the brain, often resulting in changes in behavior, movements, or consciousness.

170.   **Sepsis**: A life-threatening condition that occurs when the body's response to an infection causes inflammation throughout the body.

171.   **Shock**: A life-threatening condition in which the body's organs and tissues are not receiving enough oxygen and nutrients due to inadequate blood flow.

172.   **Somatic Pain**: Pain that originates from the skin, muscles, bones, or joints, often described as aching or throbbing.

173.   **Sputum**: Mucus that is coughed up from the lower airways, often used for diagnostic purposes in respiratory conditions.

174.   **Stoma**: An opening created surgically on the surface of the body to allow for the drainage of waste, such as in a colostomy or ileostomy.

175.   **Stridor**: A high-pitched wheezing sound often heard when breathing in, indicating a blockage or narrowing of the upper airway.

176.   **Syncope**: A temporary loss of consciousness caused by a sudden decrease in blood flow to the brain, also known as fainting.

177.   **Tachypnea**: Abnormally rapid breathing, often seen in conditions such as pneumonia or anxiety.

178.   **Thrombophlebitis**: Inflammation of a vein that is associated with the formation of a blood clot.

179.   **Vasodilation**: The widening of blood vessels, which increases blood flow and decreases blood pressure.

180.   **Analgesic**: A medication that relieves pain.

181.   **Auscultate**: To listen to sounds within the body, typically using a stethoscope.

182.   **Cannula**: A flexible tube inserted into a vein or body cavity for draining fluids, administering medication, or inserting instruments.

183.   **Cholecystectomy**: Surgical removal of the gallbladder.

184.   **Comorbidity**: The presence of two or more chronic conditions in a patient.

185.   **Decubitus Ulcer**: A pressure sore or bed sore, caused by prolonged pressure on the skin.

186.   **Dilation and Curettage (D&C)**: A surgical procedure in which the cervix is dilated and the uterine lining is scraped.

187.   **Diuresis**: Increased production of urine.

188.   **Epistaxis**: Nosebleed.

189.   **Fissure**: A narrow opening or crack, especially in the skin.

190.   **Hematocrit**: The percentage of red blood cells in the blood.

191.   **Hypoxemia**: Abnormally low levels of oxygen in the blood.

192. **Lumbar Puncture**: A procedure in which a needle is inserted into the lower spine to collect cerebrospinal fluid or administer medication.

193. **Malaise**: A general feeling of discomfort or illness.

194. **Nephrectomy**: Surgical removal of a kidney.

195. **Paracentesis**: A procedure to remove fluid from the abdominal cavity.

196. **Pericarditis**: Inflammation of the pericardium, the membrane surrounding the heart.

197. **Rhonchi**: Rattling or wheezing sounds heard when listening to the chest with a stethoscope, often due to mucus in the airways.

198. **Tachycardia**: Abnormally rapid heart rate.

199. **Vasopressor**: A medication that constricts blood vessels and raises blood pressure.

200. **Anuria**: The absence of urine production or excretion.

201. **Bronchoscopy**: A procedure that allows a doctor to view the inside of the airways and lungs.

202. **Capillary Refill**: The time it takes for blood to return to the capillaries after they have been compressed, often used as a measure of circulation.

203. **Cataract**: A clouding of the lens of the eye that can impair vision.

204. **Contraindication**: A factor that makes the use of a drug or treatment inadvisable, usually because it may harm the patient.

205. **Dorsiflexion**: The movement of bending the foot or hand upwards at the ankle or wrist.

206. **Echocardiogram**: A test that uses sound waves to create images of the heart.

207. **Embolus**: A blood clot, air bubble, or other foreign material that travels through the bloodstream and lodges in a blood vessel, causing obstruction.

208. **Endocarditis**: Inflammation of the inner lining of the heart chambers and valves.

209. **Exacerbation**: A worsening or flare-up of a disease or condition.

210. **Exophthalmos**: Abnormal protrusion of the eyeball, often associated with thyroid disorders.

211. **Fibrillation**: Rapid, irregular contractions of the heart muscles, which can be life-threatening.

212. **Hematemesis**: The vomiting of blood, often due to bleeding in the digestive tract.

213. **Hyponatremia**: A lower-than-normal concentration of sodium in the blood.

214. **Ischemia**: A restriction in blood supply to tissues, causing a shortage of oxygen and glucose needed for cellular metabolism.

215. **Myopia**: Nearsightedness, a condition in which close objects are seen clearly but distant objects are blurred.

216. **Neutropenia**: A low level of neutrophils, a type of white blood cell, in the blood, which can increase the risk of infection.

217. **Oliguria**: Abnormally low urine output, often defined as less than 400 milliliters per day in adults.

218. **Paraplegia**: Paralysis of the lower half of the body, including both legs.

219. **Petechiae**: Tiny, pinpoint-sized purple or red spots on the skin caused by small amounts of bleeding under the skin.

220. **Prophylaxis**: Treatment given or action taken to prevent disease.

221. **Pulmonary Embolism**: A blockage in one of the pulmonary arteries in the lungs, usually caused by a blood clot that travels to the lungs from a vein in the leg.

222. **Purpura**: Purple or red discoloration of the skin or mucous membranes caused by bleeding underneath the skin.

223. **Retrograde**: Moving backward or against the normal direction.

224. **Scoliosis**: A sideways curvature of the spine.

225. **Sepsis**: A life-threatening condition that occurs when the body's response to an infection causes inflammation throughout the body.

226. **Sputum**: Mucus that is coughed up from the lower airways, often used for diagnostic purposes in respiratory conditions.

227. **Stenosis**: The narrowing or constriction of a body passage or opening.

228. **Stoma**: An opening created surgically on the surface of the body to allow for the drainage of waste, such as in a colostomy or ileostomy.

229. **Stridor**: A high-pitched wheezing sound often heard when breathing in, indicating a blockage or narrowing of the upper airway.

230. **Syncope**: A temporary loss of consciousness caused by a sudden decrease in blood flow to the brain, also known as fainting.

231. **Tachycardia**: Abnormally rapid heart rate.

232. **Thrombophlebitis**: Inflammation of a vein that is associated with the formation of a blood clot.

233. **Tracheostomy**: A surgical procedure to create an opening in the neck into the trachea (windpipe) to allow for breathing.

234. **Turgor**: The elasticity or resilience of the skin, often used as an indicator of hydration status.

235. **Urticaria**: Hives, a skin rash characterized by raised, red, itchy welts.

236. **Vasodilation**: The widening of blood vessels, which increases blood flow and decreases blood pressure.

237. **Ventricular Fibrillation**: A life-threatening arrhythmia (irregular heart rhythm) that can lead to cardiac arrest.

238. **Xerostomia**: Dryness of the mouth caused by reduced saliva production.

239. **Zygomatic**: Relating to the cheekbone or the area near the cheekbone.

240. **Anoxia**: A condition characterized by a severe lack of oxygen reaching the body's tissues.

241. **Ascites**: The accumulation of fluid in the abdominal cavity, often seen in patients with liver disease.

242.   **Atelectasis**: The collapse or closure of a lung or part of a lung, resulting in reduced or absent gas exchange.

243.   **Avulsion**: The tearing away of a body structure or part, often used to describe a type of injury.

244.   **Barotrauma**: Physical injury to body tissues caused by a difference in pressure between an air space inside or beside the body and the surrounding gas or fluid.

245.   **Borborygmi**: The rumbling or gurgling noise produced by the movement of gas and fluids in the intestines.

246.   **Caudal**: Toward the tail or the inferior end of the body.

247.   **Cellulitis**: A bacterial skin infection that can cause redness, swelling, and pain.

248.   **Cholecystitis**: Inflammation of the gallbladder, often due to gallstones.

249.   **Contusion**: A bruise, typically caused by a blow to the body that damages blood vessels and causes blood to leak into surrounding tissues.

250.   **Crepitus**: A crackling or grating sound or sensation produced by the rubbing together of bone fragments or irregular cartilage surfaces in a joint.

251.   **Cyanosis**: A bluish discoloration of the skin and mucous membranes caused by a lack of oxygen in the blood.

252.   **Debridement**: The removal of dead or damaged tissue from a wound to promote healing.

253.   **Dysphonia**: Difficulty speaking due to hoarseness or other vocal problems.

254. **Ecchymosis**: A discoloration of the skin resulting from bleeding underneath, typically caused by bruising.

255. **Emphysema**: A chronic lung condition characterized by shortness of breath and damage to the air sacs in the lungs.

256. **Epistaxis**: Nosebleed.

257. **Evisceration**: The displacement of organs outside of the body, often due to a traumatic injury.

258. **Hematemesis**: The vomiting of blood, often due to bleeding in the digestive tract.

259. **Hemothorax**: A collection of blood in the space between the chest wall and the lung, usually caused by injury or trauma.

260. **Hydrocephalus**: A condition characterized by the accumulation of cerebrospinal fluid in the brain, leading to increased pressure inside the skull.

261. **Hypercapnia**: Excess carbon dioxide in the bloodstream, often due to inadequate ventilation or respiratory failure.

262. **Hypertrophy**: The enlargement or overgrowth of an organ or tissue due to an increase in the size of its cells.

263. **Icterus**: Another term for jaundice, a yellowing of the skin and eyes due to a buildup of bilirubin in the blood.

264. **Incontinence**: The inability to control bowel or bladder function, leading to involuntary loss of urine or feces.

265. **Infarction**: The death of tissue or organ cells due to a lack of blood supply, often caused by a blood clot or blockage.

266. **Intussusception**: A serious condition in which one part of the intestine slides into another, causing a blockage.

267.   **Kyphosis**: Abnormal curvature of the spine, causing a hunchback or rounded back appearance.

268.   **Laryngectomy**: Surgical removal of the larynx (voice box).

269.   **Macule**: A flat, discolored spot on the skin, such as a freckle or birthmark.

270.   **Mastectomy**: Surgical removal of one or both breasts, usually to treat or prevent breast cancer.

271.   **Melanoma**: A type of skin cancer that develops from melanocytes, the cells that produce pigment in the skin.

272.   **Meningitis**: Inflammation of the meninges, the membranes that cover the brain and spinal cord, usually caused by infection.

273.   **Myalgia**: Muscular pain or tenderness, often caused by overuse or injury.

274.   **Necrosis**: The death of cells or tissues due to disease, injury, or lack of blood supply.

275.   **Nephritis**: Inflammation of the kidneys, often caused by infection or autoimmune disease.

276.   **Neurogenic**: Caused by or relating to a disorder of the nervous system.

277.   **Occlusive**: Causing or tending to cause blockage or obstruction, often used to describe a dressing or bandage.

278.   **Osteoporosis**: A condition characterized by a decrease in bone density, leading to an increased risk of fractures.

279.   **Pallor**: Unusual paleness of the skin, often a sign of illness or shock.

280.   **Perfusion**: The process of delivering blood to a capillary bed in tissue.

281.   **Petechiae**: Tiny, pinpoint, flat, red spots under the skin surface caused by bleeding.

282.   **Pneumothorax**: Air in the pleural space causing lung collapse.

283.   **Pruritus**: Itching of the skin.

284.   **Purulent**: Containing pus.

285.   **Pyelonephritis**: Inflammation of the kidney tissue, calyces, and pelvis caused by bacterial infection.

286.   **Rhinorrhea**: Thin, watery discharge from the nose (runny nose).

287.   **Sepsis**: A life-threatening condition caused by the body's response to an infection.

288.   **Sputum**: Mucus coughed up from the lower airways.

289.   **Stomatitis**: Inflammation of the mucous lining of any of the structures in the mouth.

290.   **Tachycardia**: Abnormally rapid heart rate.

291.   **Thrombophlebitis**: Inflammation of a vein caused by a blood clot.

292.   **Tinnitus**: Ringing or buzzing noise in the ears.

293.   **Torsion**: The twisting of a bodily organ on its own axis (e.g., testicular torsion).

294.   **Tracheostomy**: Surgical creation of an opening into the trachea through the neck.

295. **Urethritis**: Inflammation of the urethra, the tube that carries urine from the bladder to outside the body.

296. **Varicella**: Chickenpox, a highly contagious viral infection.

297. **Varicosity**: A varicose or permanently dilated vein.

298. **Vesicle**: A small fluid-filled blister.

299. **Xeroderma**: Abnormal dryness of the skin, mucous membranes, or conjunctiva.

300. **Acute**: Refers to a disease or condition that has a rapid onset and a short duration.

301. **Adverse Reaction**: An unexpected or harmful reaction to a medication or treatment.

302. **Alopecia**: Hair loss, often due to medical treatments, such as chemotherapy.

303. **Anemia**: A condition characterized by a deficiency of red blood cells or hemoglobin in the blood, leading to reduced oxygen transport.

304. **Anorexia**: Loss of appetite or an inability to eat.

305. **Antibiotic**: A medication used to treat bacterial infections.

306. **Anticoagulant**: A medication that prevents the formation of blood clots.

307. **Arrhythmia**: Abnormal heart rhythm, which can be too fast, too slow, or irregular.

308. **Aseptic Technique**: A method used to prevent contamination and maintain sterility, often used during medical procedures.

309. **Atherosclerosis**: A condition characterized by the buildup of plaque in the arteries, leading to reduced blood flow.

310. **Bacteriuria**: The presence of bacteria in the urine, often indicating a urinary tract infection.

311. **Bronchitis**: Inflammation of the bronchial tubes, often causing coughing and difficulty breathing.

312. **Catheter**: A flexible tube inserted into the body to drain fluids or administer medications.

313. **Catheterization**: The process of inserting a catheter into the body.

314. **Chronic**: Refers to a disease or condition that persists over a long period of time.

315. **Cirrhosis**: Scarring of the liver, often caused by long-term liver damage.

316. **Cystitis**: Inflammation of the bladder, often caused by a bacterial infection.

317. **Dehydration**: A condition characterized by a lack of adequate fluid in the body.

318. **Dementia**: A decline in cognitive function that interferes with daily life and activities.

319. **Diabetes Mellitus**: A chronic condition characterized by high blood sugar levels, often due to insufficient insulin production or insulin resistance.

320. **Dialysis**: A medical procedure used to remove waste products and excess fluids from the blood when the kidneys are unable to do so.

321.   **Dysphagia**: Difficulty or discomfort in swallowing, often due to a medical condition or injury.

322.   **Edema**: Swelling caused by excess fluid trapped in body tissues, often seen in the legs, ankles, and feet.

323.   **Emesis**: The act of vomiting or the material that is vomited.

324.   **Erythema**: Redness of the skin, often caused by inflammation or infection.

325.   **Exacerbation**: A worsening or flare-up of a disease or condition.

326.   **Exudate**: Fluid, such as pus or serum, that leaks out of blood vessels into nearby tissues due to inflammation or injury.

327.   **Fecal Incontinence**: Inability to control bowel movements, leading to involuntary passage of stool.

328.   **Fissure**: A narrow opening or crack, especially in the skin.

329.   **Flatus**: Gas in the digestive tract, expelled through the anus.

330.   **Gastritis**: Inflammation of the lining of the stomach, often causing nausea, vomiting, and abdominal pain.

331.   **Gingivitis**: Inflammation of the gums, often caused by plaque buildup.

332.   **Hemiplegia**: Paralysis of one side of the body, usually caused by a stroke or brain injury.

333.   **Hemorrhage**: Excessive bleeding, either internal or external.

334.   **Hepatitis**: Inflammation of the liver, often caused by a viral infection.

335.   **Hyperglycemia**: High blood sugar levels, often seen in patients with diabetes.

336.   **Hypoglycemia**: Low blood sugar levels, which can cause symptoms such as dizziness, confusion, and sweating.

337.   **Hypotension**: Low blood pressure, which can cause symptoms such as dizziness, fainting, and fatigue.

338.   **Incontinence**: Inability to control bladder or bowel function, leading to involuntary leakage of urine or feces.

339.   **Infarction**: Death of tissue due to lack of blood supply, often caused by a blood clot or blockage.

340.   **Ischemia**: A restriction in blood supply to tissues, causing a shortage of oxygen and glucose needed for cellular metabolism.

341.   **Jaundice**: Yellowing of the skin and whites of the eyes, usually due to liver disease or obstruction of the bile duct.

342.   **Lethargy**: A state of tiredness, lack of energy, or enthusiasm.

343.   **Lymphadenopathy**: Swollen or enlarged lymph nodes, often due to infection, inflammation, or cancer.

344.   **Malaise**: A general feeling of discomfort, illness, or unease, often the first sign of an infection or other disease.

345.   **Meningitis**: Inflammation of the meninges, the membranes surrounding the brain and spinal cord, usually caused by an infection.

346.   **Nasogastric Tube (NG Tube)**: A tube inserted through the nose and down into the stomach to provide nutrition, medication, or to remove gastric contents.

347.   **Neonate**: A newborn baby, usually up to 28 days old.

348. **Nystagmus**: Involuntary, rapid eye movements, often associated with neurological disorders or inner ear problems.

349. **Orthostatic Hypotension**: A sudden drop in blood pressure that occurs when a person stands up from a sitting or lying position.

350. **Otitis Media**: Inflammation of the middle ear, often characterized by ear pain, fever, and hearing loss.

351. **Palliative Care**: Medical care focused on providing relief from the symptoms and stress of a serious illness, rather than curing the illness itself.

352. **Paroxysmal**: Occurring suddenly and uncontrollably, often referring to a sudden onset of symptoms or a sudden attack of a disease.

353. **Pericarditis**: Inflammation of the pericardium, the sac-like membrane surrounding the heart.

354. **Pneumonia**: Inflammation of the lungs, usually caused by infection, leading to symptoms such as cough, fever, and difficulty breathing.

355. **Polypharmacy**: The use of multiple medications by a patient, often leading to potential drug interactions and side effects.

356. **Presbyopia**: Age-related loss of the ability to focus on close objects, often resulting in the need for reading glasses.

357. **Purpura**: Purple or red discoloration of the skin caused by bleeding into the skin, mucous membranes, or organs.

358. **Rhonchi**: Rattling or wheezing sounds heard when listening to the chest, often due to mucus in the airways.

359. **Splenomegaly**: Enlargement of the spleen, often due to infection, inflammation, or other underlying conditions.

360.	**Aphasia**: A condition that affects a person's ability to communicate, often caused by a stroke or brain injury.

361.	**Aspiration**: Inhaling food, liquid, or foreign material into the lungs, which can lead to pneumonia.

362.	**Atelectasis**: Collapse or closure of a lung or part of a lung, resulting in reduced or absent gas exchange.

363.	**Axilla**: The armpit.

364.	**Bilateral**: Affecting both sides.

365.	**Bradycardia**: Abnormally slow heart rate.

366.	**Bronchodilator**: A medication that relaxes and widens the airways, making it easier to breathe.

367.	**Cachexia**: Weakness and wasting of the body due to severe illness.

368.	**Cardiopulmonary Resuscitation (CPR)**: Emergency procedure to manually pump blood and oxygen to the brain and other vital organs when the heart has stopped beating or is too weak to circulate blood effectively.

369.	**Cervical**: Relating to the neck or the uppermost part of the spine.

370.	**Circumduction**: Circular movement of a limb.

371.	**Colostomy**: Surgical procedure that brings one end of the large intestine out through the abdominal wall, creating a stoma for the passage of stool.

372.	**Craniotomy**: Surgical procedure in which a portion of the skull is removed to access the brain.

373.   **Cyanotic**: Bluish discoloration of the skin or mucous membranes due to insufficient oxygen in the blood.

374.   **Decubitus Ulcer**: A pressure sore or bed sore, caused by prolonged pressure on the skin.

375.   **Diaphoresis**: Excessive sweating, often due to a medical condition or as a side effect of medication.

376.   **Dyspnea**: Difficulty breathing, often described as shortness of breath or breathlessness.

377.   **Ecchymosis**: A discoloration of the skin resulting from bleeding underneath, typically caused by bruising.

378.   **Embolism**: A blood clot, air bubble, or other material that travels through the bloodstream and blocks a blood vessel.

379.   **Endocarditis**: Inflammation of the inner lining of the heart chambers and valves, often caused by infection.

380.   **Epistaxis**: Nosebleed.

381.   **Erythematous**: Redness of the skin or mucous membranes due to dilation and congestion of superficial capillaries.

382.   **Foley Catheter**: A type of indwelling urinary catheter that is held in place by a balloon filled with sterile water.

383.   **Glasgow Coma Scale**: A neurological scale used to assess the level of consciousness in patients with brain injuries.

384.   **Hematoma**: A localized collection of blood outside the blood vessels, usually in liquid form within the tissue.

385.   **Hypertonic**: Having a higher osmotic pressure than another solution.

386.   **Integumentary System**: The organ system that protects the body from various kinds of damage.

387.   **Lymphedema**: Swelling (usually in the legs or arms) caused by the retention of lymphatic fluid due to blockage or removal of lymph nodes.

388.   **Narcotic**: A drug that relieves pain and induces sleep.

389.   **Nystatin**: An antifungal medication used to treat fungal infections, such as oral thrush or yeast infections.

390.   **Orthostatic Hypotension**: A sudden drop in blood pressure that occurs when a person stands up from a sitting or lying position.

391.   **Osmosis**: The movement of solvent molecules through a semipermeable membrane into a region of higher solute concentration, equalizing the concentrations on each side of the membrane.

392.   **Ostomy**: A surgical procedure to create an opening (stoma) from an area inside the body to the outside.

393.   **Paralysis**: Loss of muscle function in part of your body. It can be localized or generalized, partial or complete, and temporary or permanent.

394.   **Paresthesia**: An abnormal sensation, typically tingling or pricking ("pins and needles"), caused chiefly by pressure on or damage to peripheral nerves.

395.   **Pericardial Effusion**: An abnormal accumulation of fluid in the pericardial cavity, the sac around the heart.

396.   **Peripheral Vascular Disease (PVD)**: A circulatory condition in which narrowed blood vessels reduce blood flow to the limbs.

397.   **Phlebitis**: Inflammation of a vein, usually in the legs.

398. **Plasma**: The liquid component of blood, in which the blood cells are suspended.

399. **Pleural Effusion**: An abnormal accumulation of fluid in the pleural space, the space between the lungs and the chest wall.

400. **Pneumothorax**: A collapsed lung that occurs when air leaks into the space between the lung and chest wall.

401. **Polypharmacy**: The use of multiple medications by a patient, often associated with increased risk of adverse effects.

402. **Postprandial**: After a meal.

403. **Presbycusis**: Age-related hearing loss.

404. **Prophylaxis**: Treatment given or action taken to prevent disease.

405. **Pruritus**: Itching of the skin, often due to skin conditions or allergies.

406. **Pulmonary Edema**: Fluid accumulation in the lungs, often due to heart failure.

407. **Pulmonary Embolism**: Blockage of a pulmonary artery by a blood clot, which can be life-threatening.

408. **Purulent**: Containing pus, often a sign of infection.

409. **Quadriplegia**: Paralysis of all four limbs and usually the trunk, caused by injury to the spinal cord in the cervical spine.

410. **Respite Care**: Short-term care provided to relieve caregivers, often for a few hours or days.

411. **Sclerotherapy**: Treatment for varicose veins or hemorrhoids that involves injecting a solution to shrink the vein.

412.   **Sepsis**: A life-threatening condition caused by the body's response to an infection, which can lead to organ failure.

413.   **Serous**: Thin, watery fluid, often used to describe certain types of body fluids.

414.   **Stenosis**: Abnormal narrowing of a body opening or passageway.

415.   **Suppository**: A solid medication that is inserted into the rectum, vagina, or urethra, where it dissolves or melts to release the medication.

416.   **Thrombophlebitis**: Inflammation of a vein caused by a blood clot.

417.   **Tracheostomy**: Surgical creation of an opening in the trachea (windpipe) to assist with breathing.

418.   **Urticaria**: Hives, a skin rash characterized by itchy, raised welts.

419.   **Varicosity**: The condition of being varicose, often referring to enlarged or twisted veins.

420.   **Vasodilation**: The widening of blood vessels, which results in increased blood flow.

421.   **Xerostomia**: Dry mouth, often caused by reduced saliva production.

422.   **Afebrile**: Without fever.

423.   **Anuria**: Absence of urine production.

424.   **Apnea**: Temporary cessation of breathing.

425.   **Asepsis**: Absence of pathogens, often achieved through sterile techniques.

426.   **Atrophy**: Wasting away or decrease in size of a body part, tissue, or organ.

427.   **Axillary**: Pertaining to the armpit.

428.   **Cachexia**: A state of ill health, wasting syndrome, and malnutrition, often associated with chronic diseases such as cancer.

429.   **Cholecystectomy**: Surgical removal of the gallbladder.

430.   **Contraindication**: A specific situation in which a drug, procedure, or surgery should not be used because it may be harmful to the patient.

431.   **Cyanosis**: A bluish discoloration of the skin and mucous membranes due to insufficient oxygen in the blood.

432.   **Dysuria**: Painful or difficult urination.

433.   **Ecchymosis**: Discoloration of the skin resulting from bleeding underneath, typically caused by bruising.

434.   **Edema**: Swelling caused by excess fluid trapped in body tissues.

435.   **Epistaxis**: Bleeding from the nose.

436.   **Erythema**: Redness of the skin caused by dilated blood vessels.

437.   **Exacerbation**: A worsening of symptoms or disease.

438.   **Exophthalmos**: Abnormal protrusion of the eyeball.

439. **Fecal Impaction**: A large, hard mass of stool that gets stuck in the rectum and cannot be expelled.

440. **Gastritis**: Inflammation of the lining of the stomach.

441. **Gastrostomy**: Surgical creation of an opening (stoma) into the stomach through the abdominal wall, usually for feeding or drainage purposes.

442. **Hematemesis**: Vomiting of blood.

443. **Hemiparesis**: Weakness on one side of the body.

444. **Hemoptysis**: Coughing up blood or bloody sputum from the respiratory tract.

445. **Hypercapnia**: Excess carbon dioxide in the bloodstream, often due to inadequate ventilation or respiratory failure.

446. **Hyperkalemia**: Elevated levels of potassium in the blood.

447. **Hypertonic**: Having a higher osmotic pressure than another solution.

448. **Hypoglycemia**: Low blood sugar, which can cause symptoms such as dizziness, sweating, and confusion.

449. **Hypotension**: Low blood pressure, which can cause symptoms such as dizziness, lightheadedness, and fainting.

450. **Ileostomy**: Surgical creation of an opening (stoma) into the ileum (the last part of the small intestine) through the abdominal wall, usually for the diversion of fecal matter.

451. **Infarction**: Tissue death (necrosis) due to a lack of blood supply.

452. **Infiltrate**: The accumulation of fluid, pus, or blood in the tissues, often seen on a chest X-ray as a white shadow.

453. **Intussusception**: The telescoping of one part of the intestine into another, causing an obstruction.

454. **Ketosis**: An abnormal increase in ketone bodies in the blood, often seen in uncontrolled diabetes or fasting.

455. **Laceration**: A deep cut or tear in the skin or flesh.

456. **Lumbar Puncture**: A procedure in which a needle is inserted into the spinal canal to collect cerebrospinal fluid or administer medications.

457. **Malabsorption**: Impaired absorption of nutrients from the gastrointestinal tract.

458. **Melena**: Black, tarry stool due to the presence of partially digested blood.

459. **Myocardial Infarction**: Heart attack, which occurs when blood flow to a part of the heart is blocked for a long enough time that part of the heart muscle is damaged or dies.

460. **Necrosis**: Death of cells or tissues due to disease, injury, or lack of blood supply.

461. **Neurogenic**: Caused by or relating to disorders of the nervous system.

462. **Occlusion**: Blockage or closure of a blood vessel or hollow organ.

463. **Ophthalmoscope**: Instrument used to examine the interior structures of the eye, including the retina and optic nerve.

464.   **Osteomyelitis**: Inflammation of the bone, usually caused by infection.

465.   **Palpation**: Examination by touch, often used to assess the size, consistency, and location of organs and tissues.

466.   **Paroxysmal**: Sudden and recurring, often referring to a sudden attack or episode of symptoms.

467.   **Peristalsis**: Wave-like contractions of the muscles in the digestive tract that move food along the digestive system.

468.   **Pharyngitis**: Inflammation of the pharynx (throat), often causing a sore throat.

469.   **Pneumonitis**: Inflammation of the lung tissue, often caused by infection or exposure to irritants.

470.   **Polyuria**: Excessive production of urine, often seen in conditions such as diabetes mellitus.

471.   **Prognosis**: The likely course or outcome of a disease or condition.

472.   **Pulmonary Function Test (PFT)**: A test that measures how well the lungs are working, including the amount of air inhaled and exhaled and how efficiently oxygen is transferred into the bloodstream.

473.   **Pyuria**: The presence of pus in the urine, often indicating a urinary tract infection.

474.   **Rales**: Abnormal crackling or rattling sounds heard when listening to the lungs, often due to fluid in the airways.

475.   **Sclera**: The tough, white outer layer of the eyeball.

476.   **Sepsis**: A life-threatening condition caused by the body's response to an infection, which can lead to organ failure.

477. **Sputum**: Mucus coughed up from the lower airways, often used for diagnostic purposes in respiratory conditions.

478. **Stoma**: An artificial opening created surgically on the surface of the body, such as in a colostomy or ileostomy, to allow for the drainage of waste.

479. **Subcutaneous**: Underneath the skin.

480. **Tachypnea**: Abnormally rapid breathing rate.

481. **Thrombocytopenia**: A condition characterized by a low platelet count in the blood, which can lead to increased risk of bleeding.

482. **Trachea**: The windpipe, which connects the larynx to the bronchi and allows air to pass to and from the lungs.

483. **Tympanic**: Relating to the eardrum or tympanic membrane.

484. **Urinary Retention**: Inability to completely empty the bladder.

485. **Vasopressor**: A medication that constricts blood vessels and increases blood pressure.

486. **Venipuncture**: The process of puncturing a vein with a needle for the purpose of drawing blood or administering medication.

487. **Vesicant**: A substance that causes blistering or severe tissue injury when it leaks from a blood vessel into surrounding tissues.

488. **Vital Signs**: Measurements of the body's basic functions, including temperature, pulse rate, respiratory rate, and blood pressure.

489. **X-ray**: A type of electromagnetic radiation used to create images of the inside of the body, especially the bones.

490. **Abduction**: Movement of a limb away from the midline of the body.

491. **Adduction**: Movement of a limb toward the midline of the body.

492. **Ambulate**: To walk or move about.

493. **Auscultation**: Listening to sounds within the body, usually with a stethoscope.

494. **Bradykinesia**: Slowness of movement.

495. **Catheterize**: To insert a catheter into a body cavity or organ.

496. **Circumduction**: Circular movement of a limb, such as the arm or leg.

497. **Crepitus**: A crackling or popping sound, often heard in joints.

498. **Dehiscence**: Separation of previously joined wound edges, often seen in surgical incisions.

499. **Dysphasia**: Difficulty speaking or understanding speech, often due to brain injury or stroke.